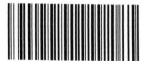

MAKING SENSE OF "IT"

MAKING SENSE OF "IT"

A GUIDE TO SEX FOR TEENS
(AND THEIR PARENTS, TOO!)

ALISON MACKLIN

VIVA
EDITIONS

Published in the United States by Viva Editions, an imprint of Start Midnight, LLC, 101 Hudson Street, Thirty-Seventh Floor, Suite 3705, Jersey City, NJ 07302.

Printed in the United States.
Cover design: Allyson Fields
Cover photograph: iStock
Interior photographs: iStock, Shutterstock
Illustrations: Sofie Birkin
Text design: Frank Wiedemann

First Edition.
10 9 8 7 6 5 4 3 2 1

Trade paper ISBN: 978-1-63228-064-0
E-book ISBN: 978-1-63228-065-7

Library of Congress Cataloging-in-Publication Data is available on file.

*This book is dedicated to
my biggest champion, Blake.*

TABLE OF CONTENTS

INTRODUCTION

Dear Teen,

So, your parent bought this book for you, huh? Don't worry. Mine did, too. I mean, not *this* book, but another book. One that was just about puberty. But for me, that was it. We didn't talk about the book, what it said, or anything. There was no conversation. There wasn't an attitude like, "Let's figure this out" or, "Hey, this is important and I am here for you." It was just a book, on my pillow when I got home from school. I remember trying to

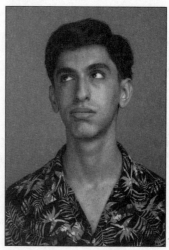

You got this book and rolled your eyes, didn't you? Simmer down and give it a chance!

talk to my mom about what I read (there was no way I was going to talk to my dad) and that experience being embarrassing and also disappointing. My mom, who was so good at talking to me about so many other things and making sure I knew I was valued and important, couldn't talk to me about sex. I guess she answered my questions about my period and sexual health (i.e. made sure I started seeing a gynecologist) but other than that? Nothing except, "Just don't do 'it.'"

I had all these questions! What did it mean to do "it"? What about masturbation, is that okay? Am I dirty for having sexual fantasies? What about kissing, is that safe? What if I touch someone's penis, can I get pregnant? Giving a blow job is safe, right? If I take the pill I am totally safe, right? If I douche after sex, I won't get pregnant, right? And forget discussing my sexual identity or who I was attracted to. I had so. Many. Questions. And I felt like I didn't have anyone to talk to. I grew up in a house where knowledge and discovery were treasured and encouraged. But in this one simple gesture, I felt like this was the one subject that I couldn't talk about. Bummer.

So, while your parents *also* went and bought this book, this book is different. It's different because it isn't meant to be the end-all, be-all about sex and sexuality. This book is meant to help you start and continue to have conversations about sex and sexuality. It's designed to ensure that the dialogue between you and your parent(s) isn't closed but always open. Because they don't have all the answers. I don't have all the answers. But I am committed to helping and honoring you wherever you are in your desire to learn about sex and sexuality. And so are your parents. We want you to have the facts. Medically accurate information that ensures you have all the information to make the best decisions for your sexual health throughout your life—whether you're 17, 25, 45 or 85 (because, yeah, even your grandparents are having sex).

1

UGH. DO WE REALLY HAVE TO TALK ABOUT *IT*?

Okay, so your parents got this book because they want you to know you can talk to them about all things sex-related. That's easy to say, but not easy to do. It's one thing to talk to your parents about reproductive anatomy or periods or even about contraception when it isn't about you. But what about when it is? And how do you begin to talk to them about your sexuality? What if your sexual identity doesn't align with your biological body parts? And how about talking to them about who you're attracted to and when you should become sexually active? Do those kinds of conversations freak you out when you think of having them with your parents? My guess is that, regardless of what kind of relationship you have with your parents, you have some anxiety around talking to them about the sex things.

Okay, here's the biggest thing to remember about talking to your parents about sex and sexuality: they are humans. That means that at one point in their lives, they probably had the same questions you do. Maybe not *exactly* the same, but no one was born knowing this information. The way your parents learned about sex might have been a great experience or it may have been not the best. But, here's the thing—they want you to know about sex so that you can make informed decisions and stay safe. They also want you to have a sexually healthy relationship when you're ready. Meaning, they know sex can be pleasurable and they want you to be able to experience that—with the right partner and at the right time.

We know talking to your parents about sex isn't easy. But why? Why is this topic so hard to talk about? Well, for one thing, it's private. It involves your "private parts," and sexual acts are something to do with a romantic partner. Sex, sexual health, sexuality—these topics aren't exactly dinner-table topics in the United States. Just so you know, there are countries out there where families do talk about sexuality at the dinner table and it is the norm, not the exception. In these countries (like Denmark, Sweden and the Netherlands) unplanned teen pregnancies are much lower. In fact, the United States has a higher rate of unplanned teen pregnancies than in most other developed countries.[1] Why do you think that is? Studies show that in addition to having high unplanned teen pregnancy rates, the United States also has higher rates of Sexually Transmitted Infections (STIs). What's the fundamental difference here? Those other countries talk about sex early and often in a way that is developmentally appropriate. That means that when a teen decides they want to have sex, they have all the facts and can make informed decisions about how to stay safe and how to advocate for themselves in a sexual relationship. So, whether your

---

[1] "Guttmacher Institute. 2001. "Differences in Teenage Pregnancy Rates Among Five Developed Countries: The Roles of Sexual Activity and Contraceptive Use." Accessed January 17, 2018. http://www.guttmacher.org/journals/psrh/2001/11/differences-teenage-pregnancy-rates-among-five-developed-countries-roles.

parents started talking to you as a young child about consent and what the right names of the body parts are or whether they are just begin-ning to, give them a break.

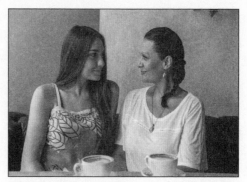

Okay, so maybe you and your mom aren't going to have this picture-perfect setting for a conversation, but the important thing is you're both making time to talk about all the things.

They *are* trying to talk about it.

Just because your parents want to talk with you about sex and sexuality doesn't mean you all have to agree on every-thing. Spoiler alert: your parents (just like you) have a lot of opinions and values about sex. So, asking your parents what they think about different things we'll talk about in this book can start the conversation. You can also figure out what they think by using the conversations starters at the end of each chapter, or by trying something more general like, "Did your parents ever talk to you about sex? What was that like?" Or how about, "I think some of my friends are having sex, and I want to know what you think about that." Or, you could try, "What's one thing you wish you knew before you started having sex?"

Remember, your parents are new to this, too. In order for them to be comfortable sharing information about their own experiences or values about sex and sexuality, they are going to want the same things you want: trust, respect, and a rela-tionship that is judgment-free. I guarantee that your parents probably have some pretty interesting experiences about their own sexual journeys. But, you need to respect their boundaries (just like they need to respect yours). There are some things that will (and should) remain private (for both of you). Just remember, your parents will appreciate your honesty and openness, just like you will appreciate theirs.

2

A FEW NOTES FOR THE PARENTS

Talking to your kids about the, um, sex stuff can be overwhelming, scary and intimidating, and sometimes feel like you're throwing spaghetti on the wall to see if it sticks. Even for those of us who do this for a living, no one feels totally prepared for the first time we are asked, "Where do babies come from?" (Especially when it happens in response to your question of whether they wanted milk or water with their dinner. . . .)

The good news? You care, and you want to do what is best for your child. That attitude alone means you have taken the first step to being an "askable adult." What's that, you say? Well, an askable adult is a person who feels comfortable with others asking them some pretty personal stuff, because they know and trust that you're going to respond to them with care, compassion and respect. That you aren't going to judge them for being curious, and you aren't going to laugh at them for asking. That's it. That's the goal. So, congratulations on taking the first step—you bought this book! And this book is filled with basic information about sex and sexuality (because they are different) that you can use to help answer your teen's questions. There are conversation-starters that can help you and your youth have meaningful discussions, and there are fun facts and myth-busters throughout. In no way is this a medical journal. Nor does it strive to be the end-all, be-all when it comes to sex and sexuality. There are lots of great resources, organizations, doctors, and nurses that can get into some of the details with you and your teen if you need it. The intent of this book is simply to help you have the important conversations that are critical to keeping your kiddo safe and healthy. And why me? Because I'm a parent, too. I just happen to be a parent who has been working as a professional in the sex education field for fourteen years who's talked to lots of parents and teens about this stuff. I am a parent who wants her kids to grow up in a society where people of every gender and orientation are treated equally. I am a parent who wants people who are having sex to be having consensual and pleasurable sex. When I started in this field, there were still a lot of scare tactics being used, like, "Look at this picture of the penis with herpes! If you don't want herpes, then don't have sex!" There was also a lot of money (both private and federal) going into programs that shamed youth for their sexual feelings, and stigmatized youth who didn't fall into traditional gender roles or heterosexual relationships. Programs that didn't account for the fact that there are people in our society who suffer from trauma both personally and historically, as well as programs that didn't account for the fact that teens are really smart and, given the facts, are perfectly capable of making decisions about their bodies.

We all start somewhere. I came into this field wanting youth to be empowered to make decisions about their sex lives, and I have dedicated my career to this purpose, working nationally with some of the smartest folks in this field and learning as much as I could. Some people know a lot about sex and sexuality, and some don't, and that's okay. I'm not going to judge, because there was a time in my life when I didn't know what I currently know, and I learn something new in this field every day. So, know you aren't alone. Know that you have resources. And know that we are all just parents trying to help our children live sexually healthy lives.

THE TALK

Here's the thing. There isn't just one talk. Sexuality should be something that is discussed often. There are so many aspects to sex. There isn't anyone in the world who can cover everything in just one talk. So, relax. These conversations don't have to cover every single thing every time the topic of sex and sexuality come up. Conversations about sex and sexuality can happen in the car, in the kitchen, on vacation, just about anywhere. They can be initiated by you, or your teen might bring up a question (or lots of questions). These are what we in the sex ed biz call "teachable moments."

A teachable moment means that the parent seizes the moment as it presents itself in a conversational and casual manner. A teachable moment gives you an opportunity to help your teen understand concepts about sexuality. For example, it may be that you and your teen are watching TV together and there is a sex scene. Rather than just ignoring it, talk about it with your teen. Ideally in that moment, but maybe for your relationship it will be better to come back to that scene at a later date. Talk with your teen about

7

whether they saw consent being asked for and given. Or whether those engaged in a sexual act used any form of protection against STIs and pregnancy (if it's heterosexual sex). If it isn't heterosexual sex, there are other opportunities for discussions. The opportunities are endless, really. But as a parent, you shouldn't feel like that one TV show sex scene is the time where you have to cram in a ton of conversation and information. Choose one or two things to focus on— it's a two-minute conversation with basic info and succinct statements.

The purpose of these teachable moments (aside from getting some info out there) is to open dialogue. Rather than criticizing the fact that the couple on the screen didn't use a condom, ask your teen something like, "I wonder if they used a condom. What do you think?" By asking your teen their thoughts you will learn a lot about their base knowledge level, what their values around different aspects of sex and sexuality are, and what they know about different sexual health concepts. Maybe your teen responds, "No, they wouldn't use a condom because condoms don't do anything." Well, then, as a parent, you have a lot of information about where your teen is, and you can make sure, either in the moment or later, to have a further conversation about the effectiveness of condoms, steps for use, why they are important, and even what impact TV shows might have on youth with regard to condom use.

Teachable moments are everywhere (not just TV). They can happen when you're listening to music together, watching a movie together, passing a billboard while driving, or talking about a friend's behavior or decision. Since just about everything can be a teachable moment, it doesn't mean you're a bad parent if you don't take advantage of each moment. That would be fairly impossible. Choose the times that fit for you and feel natural. If you present yourself as open and willing to discuss these things, your teen will often be the one who identifies the teachable moment themselves.

It's important you know what you're comfortable talking about. There might be some subjects in the realm of sexuality you're really comfortable with. Others? Not so much. You might know a lot about periods, for example, but not a lot about gender identity. And guess what? That's okay. You can't be an expert on everything. The ability of a parent to say, "I don't know" is huge. So, don't be afraid to say it. In fact, showing your teen that you don't know everything is really useful because they know it's okay if they don't know something.

If you say, "I don't know, let's look it up!" then do it.

By doing this, you're also showing your teen a few other things that are vital to having open communication about sexuality besides honesty: reliability and partnership. By the way, coming back to your teen with the correct factual answer shows you're committed to their knowledge and want them to have the right information so they can make the best decisions. Better yet, when you look up the answer together, not only are you demonstrating that you want your teen to be empowered, you're showing them legitimate sites full of medically accurate information they can reference in the future. You're showing your teen you're there for them and you're a willing partner as they try to figure out all the sex stuff. To help you both, each chapter has further informational resources you can use. Look them up together!

HOW TO KEEP YOUR COOL

The best way for a parent to avoid the deer-in-headlights, static-in-the-ears moment when presented with communicating with your teen about sex and sexuality is to know what you want to say before you find yourself in the moment. Think about your own values around issues of sex. Think about how you would respond to the following:

- How would I feel if my teen told me they are heterosexual?

- How would I feel if my teen told me they are homosexual?

- How would if feel if my teen told me they are bisexual?

- What do I think about gay marriage?

- What do I think about people who are attracted to males and females?

- If my teen was having sex, how would I feel about that?

- If I found out my teen was having sex in my house, how would I feel about that?

- How do I feel about masturbation?

- What are my thoughts about sexual assault?

- What if my teen told me they don't identify as a male but have male genitalia? (or female if they have female genitalia)

- How do I feel about my teen having a child?

- How do I feel about abortion? For me? For my teen? For my teen's partner?

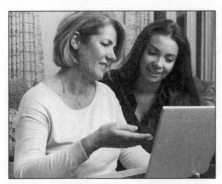

Before you start using your search engine to find the answers, I'd check out the last section of this book for reliable and teen-friendly (and let's be honest, parent-friendly) websites.

Thinking about how you feel about the above, and other situations, can help you frame your conversations with your teen. Maybe you have a value around something but don't want to impart that value on your teen. Or, maybe you want to try to ensure that your teen values the same things as you. How you respond to questions will influence your teen, so thinking about what you want that influence to be prior to getting into the conversation is critical. Perhaps you want them to know you will love and support them no matter whom they are attracted to. Or maybe you want them to have a healthy sexual relationship with their partner, but not until they are married or after a certain age. Thinking about what you want for your teen and what you value will help you be prepared for those questions and revelations when they happen. Because, let's face it, the conversations are going to happen when you least expect it. Parenting and teachable moments are rarely something you can predict!

You should also think about how much of your own experiences you want to share. Sharing personal experiences can help your teen see you as human and help normalize behavior and feelings. Throughout the book there are conversations starters, but you might not feel comfortable answering all the questions. That's okay. You're entitled to have your own boundaries when it comes to talking about your own sexuality, just like your teen. By modeling those boundaries, you're actually showing your teen solid boundary-setting they can learn from. Are some things too private to discuss? If a question comes up that you aren't comfortable answering, think about how you can make sure your teen gets the information without feeling judged or shut down.

When a teen asks you a personal question about your sexuality, it's important to think about the intent of their question. If you get a sense that the teen is trying to understand whether they are normal or not, that's one thing. If you feel like they are trying to make you feel embarrassed, or that the information they are asking isn't relevant to their learning, then don't share it. It might help for you to think about the question behind the question. Are they asking you about whether you masturbate because they *really* want to know? Are they asking because they want to know if masturbation is normal and okay to do? As a parent, you don't have to share anything about your sexuality that you don't want to. It's *your* experience, right?

When your teen asks you a question, it's going to be important to not make assumptions about behavior based on what they are asking you. If your teen is asking you about blow jobs, for example, it doesn't mean they've had one or given one. They may have heard something in school or seen something in a movie. Often teens are asking because they want to know what it is, or why someone would do it (like, why is this even a thing?), and they are asking you because they trust you to give them information or help them understand. Just because a teen is curious about something does not mean they are doing it. Remember, there is often a question behind the question. Are they trying to normalize behavior? Are they asking for clarification? Are they trying to shock you? Are they testing you? Your initial response is going to tell them a lot. If you freak out and yell and start accusing them of engaging in blow jobs, the conversation is not going to go well. By staying cool and nonjudgmental, you can ask further questions to truly get to what they are trying to understand and support them.

STAY COOL

If your teen asks you something, make sure you really understand what they are asking. It's okay to ask follow-up questions. (Asking follow-up questions not only makes sure you are speaking directly to their question, but it can buy you some extra time to figure out how to respond.) Repeating what they ask back to them ("Are you asking . . . ?") can really help make sure you're both engaging in clear communication. Additionally, by restating the question or statement, you're validating what your teen is saying. This validation is reassuring and helps your teen know they are valued.

These conversations are hard. If they were easy, you wouldn't have bought a book looking for help. Pretty much every parent struggles with talking about sex the "right" way. It's okay if you make mistakes, but try not to argue, judge, or tell them what to do. Topics

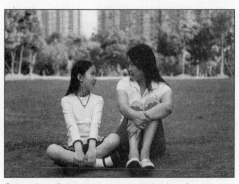

Get ready—what your teen says may shock you!

13

about sexuality are polarizing. Think about same-sex marriage. Gender-neutral bathrooms. Abortion. Everyone has an opinion. Practicing having open, honest

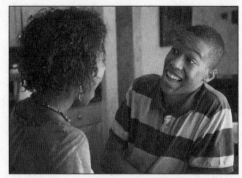

Definitely expect looks like this while you're talking with your teen.

and nonjudgmental conversations can help to ensure the lines of communication stay open. You aren't always going to agree. But you can always show each other respect.

It's important to think about your tone of voice and body language. Are you staying calm? (Take a breath and remain calm!) If you need a minute, validate what they are saying ("What a great question!") to buy yourself some time and get a hold of yourself. Are you standing with your arms crossed in a "don't talk to me" kind of way, or are you relaxed and open? What is your face doing? Are you smiling? Frowning? Surprised? Shocked? Sometimes how you communicate nonverbally can be the most impactful. If you want to make sure your teen is comfortable and talking to you openly, then make sure you are showing them you're there to talk about anything and everything, and you aren't going to judge them.

You think this whole sex convo isn't exactly a piece of cake, but think about what you were like at their age. What did you know about sex? You think *you're* nervous? They are, too! Acknowledge that this isn't easy—it's awkward. Honor the fact that they are having a hard time asking. But they *are* asking. (Major win!) Use curiosity as an opportunity to start conversations, not end them. Here are some ideas for honoring where they are and keeping the conversation going:

- "Thanks for asking that!"
- "What a great question!"
- "I'm so glad you asked me."
- "I don't know the answer, let's figure it out together."
- "It makes me feel good you are trusting me to tell me _____."
- "I remember I had a similar question when I was your age."

Remember, sarcasm and jokes aren't always helpful when you're talking about serious subjects. It can make the teen feel undervalued or criticized.

Keep your answers simple and short by using basic language and brief responses. Avoid the word vomit (where you just keep talking and talking, and the more you talk, the more confusing things become).

Always try to respond. It might not be the most ideal time, or you may not have your answer ready, but if you validate what they are saying as important and make a plan to get back to it, you aren't avoiding the question and you're still keeping the door open for future conversations. (Just make sure you actually come back to it when the time is right.)

THINGS TO REMEMBER WHEN HAVING CONVERSATIONS ABOUT SEX:

Assure and affirm. Make sure your teen knows you're grateful they are asking you questions and sharing opinions. They've taken a risk and made themselves vulnerable. Saying something like, "Thanks for asking that!" or, "I'm really glad you asked me/want to talk about that," can go a long way to making your teen feel safe in coming to you about topics of sex and sexuality.

Respond with empathy. It isn't easy to talk about sex and sexuality, so acknowledge that these conversations are hard and try to understand things from their perspective.

Don't be afraid to not know the answer. It's okay to say "I don't know." It's also okay to need time to think about something and check your resources to make sure you have an informed response.

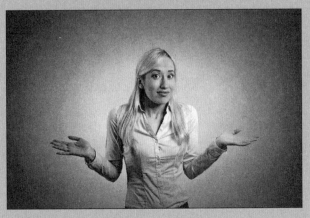

It's okay to not know!

3

HOW TEENS AND PARENTS SHOULD USE THIS BOOK

Okay, now that you know a little bit about the intent behind this book, let's talk about the most effective way to use the information in the book: any way that works for you! Some people like to read front-to-back and go through every activity and check out each additional resource. But that isn't the only way the book can be used, and coincidently, just like sexuality, there isn't one right way to go about learning the information. So, if you're interested in using the book as a reference, go for it! If you would like to skip around to topic areas that are the most useful, that's an option too. What you're going to discover, if you don't already know, is that sex and sexuality have a lot of overlap and topic areas can go in many different directions. I've organized topics in ways I think make sense, and I reference other parts of the book when there is overlap so that it's as user-friendly as possible.

This book was written with the audience of teens in mind. When I am categorizing teens, I mean anyone who is 13–19, or 8th grade and older. I use medically accurate terms and information and nationally informed guidelines for developmental appropriateness. However, every person is different. Parents: it's going to be up to you to determine whether or not the content is appropriate for your youth.

Also, parents, while I've got your attention, you should not only think about whether your teen is ready for the content, but whether you have ever talked about sex with your teen before this. How much have you talked? What do you know (and what *don't* you know)? What is your teen's level of maturity? Do you use medically accurate terminology for private parts in your family? Some youth who are younger than 13 may be ready to have these conversations. Others may not. Some youth may be ready to have conversations about some of the topics in the book, but not ready for others. As a parent, you get to decide.

The only requirement I have for both of you as you use this book is to practice respect. Yeah, sure, it might be embarrassing to talk about some of these topics, or you might have different opinions about what you read. So, it's important for you to have respect for each other, share only what feels comfortable, and also to respect each other if you have different opinions. To help guide conversations, at the end of each chapter, you will see a set of questions teens can ask parents and vice versa. I encourage you to go over the questions together, though, because this is really the best opportunity for both of you to have some pretty awesome, open conversations. If you aren't sure about having a face-to-face convo, there are other ways to get a dialogue going. A friend of mine bought a journal to share with her daughter. In it they answer the conversation questions posed at the end of each section and trade it back and forth. They also open it up for other questions because, well, in this biz answering questions often leads to more questions! For my friend and her daughter, this is a more comfortable way for them to have really important discussions, and it allows for both the parent and the teen to make sure they are stating their thoughts, questions and ideas in ways that are respectful. This is just another idea. How you decide to have the conversation is up to you.

Give yourselves a pat on the back. You're opening the door for interesting and fun (and sometimes funny) conversations. Relax and roll with it—it's going to be great.

Enjoy!

4

IT'S SCIENCE!

A SUPER QUICK DIVE INTO THE TEEN BRAIN

Okay, let's be clear: I am nowhere near being a brain scientist (and yes, that's the technical name for it). But I do know a few things about the brain's development during the teen years, and I am going to briefly go over what I know. Knowing this can help frame why teens do what they do and think how they think with regards to sex.

As with the rest of the body, the brain develops as you age. The teen brain doesn't work the same as an adult brain. It also doesn't work the same as a ten-year-old's brain. So, let's take a look at the teen brain so you have a better idea of what's going on in there and why teens make decisions the way they do and act the way they do.

Let's start with the teeny, tiny pituitary gland. For such a small part of the brain, it sure does play a big role in the development of a teenager! The pituitary gland is about the size of a pea. Its job is to regulate the body's functions, especially the function of the hormone-secreting glands. So in a female-bodied person, the pituitary gland supports the operation of the ovaries, and in a male-bodied person, the pituitary gland supports the operation of the testes. Therefore, by default, the pituitary gland is responsible for sexual maturation and reproduction (to name a few things). If there is something wrong with a person's pituitary gland, it may affect how that person experiences puberty. While it's the hormones released from the ovaries or testes that are responsible for growing breasts (female-bodied) or deepening a voice (male-bodied), without the pituitary gland telling them to do their jobs, they can't.

Okay, moving on (see, I told you this was fast!). Let's talk about the hippocampus. The job of the hippocampus is to regulate emotions. It also stores memories like facts and events. It has nothing to do with short-term memory, though. This is the part of the brain that can be most damaged by alcohol use in the teenage years. Because, like with everything, it's still developing, and research shows that those who drink alcohol as a teenager show the most damage in this part of the brain as adults.[2]

The hypothalamus also produces hormones. The hormones produced in this part of the brain determine a bunch of different behavioral functions, like whether a person is hungry, sleepy, or thirsty, and even impact a person's sex drive. It also impacts a person's mood. The amount and timing of the release of these hormones dictate certain behaviors. For instance, you might notice that you feel hungry around certain times of the day. You can thank your hypothalamus for that!

---

2   White, A. M., and H. S. Swartzwelder. June 2004. "Hippocampal function during adolescence: a unique target of ethanol effects." Annals of the New York Academy of Sciences. Accessed January 17, 2018. http://www.ncbi.nlm.nih.gov/pubmed/15251891.

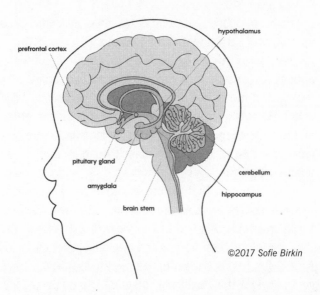

©2017 Sofie Birkin

On to the cerebellum, which is a really important part of your brain. It contains about half of the brain's neurons.[3] Your neurons are what help you function and control your body. So the fact that you can throw a ball is due to the cerebellum. By practicing your throwing so that you work on fine-tuning your skill, you will notice that you actually get better at hitting your target. Hitting your target becomes the norm, and it's a result of developing your neurons over time to ensure your body behaves in the way you're asking it to. Do you ever notice how your body doesn't quite do what you want it to as you're going through puberty? How things that used to be easy for you to control aren't anymore? Your brain has to learn to incorporate your bigger feet or the fact that you have an additional six inches in height. Due to spurts

---

3   Healthline. March 05, 2015. "Cerebellum Function, Anatomy & Definition | Body Maps." Accessed January 17, 2018. http://www.healthline.com/human-body-maps/cerebellum.

of growth in puberty, your body becomes awkward because you have to learn how to incorporate the new growth.

Now on to the amygdala. This is the middle of the brain and it's responsible for emotions. Happy, sad, angry—all the feelings. In the teen brain, this is the first part to fully develop. What that means is that teens are capable of having all the feelings that adults have. (Which can be challenging when the rest of their brain hasn't quite caught up to the emotional part.)

It also means that emotions are a huge guiding force when it comes to making decisions. Like when teens are trying to decide what to say or how to act, the first place they get information from is the emotional part of the brain. As a result, teens have a hard time thinking about the consequences of their behavior. Instead, the emotion they are feeling can dominate their decision-making process. This is amplified in an emotional situation, like a sexual situation, or a situation where they have a crush or are romantically involved with another person. Since this part of the brain is so dominant during the teen years, it can crowd out some of the more rational parts of the brain, especially when it comes to love.

The last part of the brain I want to point out is the front part, or the prefrontal cortex. This is the last part of the human brain to develop (and actually doesn't finish developing until a person is around twenty-five years old). This part of the brain is in charge of guiding emotions. It's the part of the brain that rationalizes situations and helps the individual understand the positives and negatives of different decisions. The prefrontal cortex is the part of the brain that helps a person think through all the consequences of behavior. It's also responsible for a person's ability to control themselves.

See the problem? The different parts of teens' brains aren't maturing at the same time. Which is part of why the teen years are so challenging. Teens have all these emotions happening. All. The. Time. And the feelings are strong. Sadness is *really* sad. Happiness is *really* happy. This is one of the reasons why a lot of teens struggle with depression or other forms of mental illness. The skills to cope with these immense, intense feelings haven't been developed yet.

In addition to having all these feelings, parents, teachers, bosses, friends, media, etc. are all influencing teens while they are working on developing the prefrontal cortex (the decision-making part of the brain). It can be pretty confusing! That's why there are different activities and conversation starters throughout this book. They can be used to help you practice working through different situations, and process through mistakes and successes with someone you trust.

5

WHAT DOES SEXUALITY MEAN?[4]

A GENERAL UNDERSTANDING OF SEX AND SEXUALITY AND HOW THEY ARE DIFFERENT (AND THE SAME)

Often you will hear the terms *sex* and *sexuality* used interchangeably, when they are actually different. The word *sex*, while used in many different ways, really refers to the physical act of sex. Any kind of actual sex. But the term *sexuality* encompasses everything (including sex): who you're attracted to, what kind of sex you like to have, which gender you identify with. Why is this important? Because in order to make informed decisions about your life, everyone should be familiar with not just the Ps and Vs (penises and vaginas) but everything else that goes with it. Every human being is complex, and sexuality is no different. Sexuality influences so much of our lives. Societal norms are based on sexuality. Marketing is based on sexuality. Which bathroom a person

---

4   Hunter-Geboy, Carol. *Life Planning Education: A Youth Development Program*. Washington, D.C. (1025 Vermont Ave., N.W., Suite 200, Washington 20005): Advocates for Youth, 1995.

uses is based on sexuality. Sexuality is part of our lives all day, every day. That is why it's so important to be comfortable talking about it.

To help us understand all the intricate components of sexuality, let's take a look at what are called "The Circles of Sexuality." (Shout out to Dennis M. Dailey, Professor Emeritus, University of Kansas for coming up with this concept!) This way of explaining sexuality has been around for a while. I like it because it's a good visual representation of the different concepts that make up what sexuality is, and it explains how they are interrelated. (As you read through what each circle represents, you're definitely going to see some overlap and similar concepts popping up.) Take a look at this visual representation of the Circle of Sexuality:

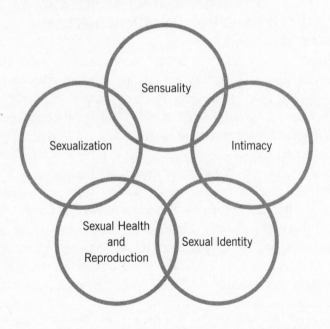

Let's dive into what concepts fit into each circle. We'll start at the top with Sensuality.

CIRCLE ONE: SENSUALITY

Sensuality is what you usually think of as "sexy." Have you ever looked in the mirror at yourself and thought, *Damn, I look good!* Or have you ever seen someone walking down the street and thought to yourself, *Whoa, they're hot!* Sensuality is when you feel like you look *good.* Or when you think someone else is *on point.* It's how you feel about your body and other people's bodies. What you find pleasurable to look at has a lot to do with how your brain interprets what you see. It also has to do with how you want to give pleasure to others. Do you find it sexy to kiss someone's neck? Or what about touching their body? Maybe that's what you like and what turns you on. Sensuality affects how we act sexually. It refers to the behaviors we like to do sexually, what things other people do that arouse us and turn us on. It refers to how we want to be touched and what stimulates the senses. It also relates to self-esteem, or how we feel about our own bodies and our ability to give and receive pleasure. For example, if we have low self-esteem we may not feel that other people will be attracted to us. Or maybe we fear that another person won't find our necks sexy enough to kiss.

Body Image

Body image is how you see yourself and your concept of worth as tied to your physical body. It's influenced by all sorts of things: messages you get from family and friends, from media and advertising, and from your partner. Think about the last time you looked in the mirror. How did you feel when you saw yourself? Proud? Attractive? Why or why not? How you feel about your body is a direct result of this idea of sensuality.

Your opinions about your body are shaped by what's around you, maybe an image of someone you saw on Instagram. You may see the image of a certain person and think, "I need to look like them in order to be considered sexy and attractive!" Or, "I'll be attractive if I wear the same kind of clothes or makeup." Or, "If I just worked out a little more or dieted more..." Comparing your body to someone who is famous because of how their body looks is often setting yourself up to be disappointed. Similarly, if you aren't seeing someone who looks like you in the movies or TV shows you watch, you might start thinking you're not attractive. Believing that you need to look a certain way to be attractive to another person puts the primary influence on what's visible from the outside and isn't a true representation for who you are. (BTW, you are beautiful the way you are!)

Pleasure

Humans determine what is pleasurable based on their senses. All of the senses: sight, hearing, touch, smell, and taste. Think about things you find pleasurable that aren't sexual. You have certain scents you like, right? You get pleasure from them? What about tastes? Think of what you eat that gives you pleasure. What about touch? What feels good when you touch it, or when someone or something touches you in a certain way? What sort of things do you see that give you pleasure? Sure, those things might not be what gives you sexual pleasure, but they make you happy. Guess what, kiddo, that joy you feel? That pleasure? Those things you like are what you find "sensual." Sensuality is what allows you to enjoy that particular scent (or taste, touch, visual, or sound).

What's a fetish? A fetish is when a person is overly attracted to or turned on by a certain thing. Not everyone has a fetish. Most people find a combination of things sensual. Someone who has a fetish has an increased sexual relationship with a certain thing. So, for example, there are people who have a "plushie" fetish. This means that they are especially attracted to people who dress up in a soft costume. They find the look of the costume as well as the feel of the costume extremely sensual and someone wearing the costume especially sexy.

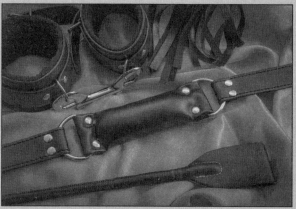

These are some examples of items that can be used in BDS&M. Practicing BDS&M means different things for different people. If you're curious about learning more about BDS&M you can go to this website: www.bettersexed. org. Just remember (and this is important!), if you want to try out BDS&M with a partner, both partners must agree to what is going to be done and when and how. This is called "consent" and we will go into this in more depth in chapter 16. BDS&M (or any other fetishized sex act) is never to be done without the other person's enthusiastic consent.

Some people cannot have sexual pleasure without their fetish, while others don't need it to have sexual pleasure, but the fetish adds to their sexual pleasure.

There are tons of sexual fetishes out there. BDS&M (Bondage and Discipline/Sadism and Masochism) is a type of fetish that involves role play and submission. It's important to remember that engaging in a fetish must always be consensual. Acting on non-consensual fetishes is illegal.

Sensuality can also refer to when you experience pleasure (taste, touch, visual, or sound) in a sexual way. Like, it turns you on, or "puts you in *the* mood." Most commonly, sensuality is thought of as meaning sexually pleasing, and can also be referred to as "erotic."

Sensuality looks different for everyone. You may really like a certain perfume or cologne, or maybe you find the taste of cigarettes on someone's breath a real "turn-off." You will discover, over time, that you learn what you find sensual and what you don't. You might also find that these things change over time. This is very normal and happens to just about everyone.

Satisfying the need for touch

All humans have a need to be touched by others who love and care about them. When you were a little kid, you probably got a lot of hugs and caring touch. Do you remember asking to be held? Or climbing onto your parents' laps for a cuddle? As you get older, this likely doesn't happen as much. First of all, you are probably too big to be held, but you're getting your need to touch satisfied in other ways. You might cuddle with your cat or hug a friend when you see them—even giving a high-five and shoulder bump is a form of touch that helps connect you with another person and fulfills that need to touch.

However, you might find that your need for touch isn't being satisfied. Or, that you're craving a type of touch that you haven't had before that you might get from a roman-

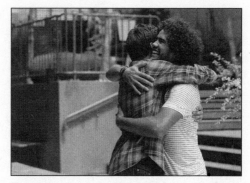

These dudes are enthusiastically hugging each other. Make sure your touches are also enthusiastically wanted!

tic partner. You may find that your craving to be touched looks different as you get older and sometimes that need to be touched could be sexual. Before you satisfy that need with another person though, you need to ask for consent. You can't just walk up to someone and hug them or touch them without them saying that's okay. Everybody's body is their own, and you need to respect that just because you have the need to be touched, the other person may not. We are going to dive into consent pretty deeply in chapter 16. You definitely want to check it out.

Feeling Attracted to Someone

Did you know that a human's brain is actually the most important "sex organ"? The brain decides who you are and are not attracted to. This isn't a choice, it's wired into who you are. Think about the senses: when you sense something, a message is sent to your brain. You then have an automated response as to whether you find pleasure in that thing. You didn't choose the fact that you have pleasure in it. Sure, you may come to like something over time, but if you don't like something? You know that pretty strongly. Right away.

When you're attracted to a certain type of person, you don't get to choose that. Being attracted to someone sexually is not a choice. Only you know who you like, and this isn't something that develops over time. Some people identify as male and are attracted to females (and vice versa), which is called heterosexuality. Some people identify as male and are attracted to males (or female attracted to females), which is homosexuality. And some people are attracted to both females and males (bisexuality), or not really attracted to anyone (asexuality). People fall all over this continuum of attraction. There isn't one right way to be, and no one chooses to be heterosexual or homosexual or bisexual or asexual. And no matter what people tell you, science says that we are born being attracted to whom we are attracted to. For more on attraction and GLB+ (Gay, Lesbian, Bisexual, +) go to chapter 9.

Fantasy

Those dreams you're having (whether you're awake or asleep)? Totally normal. They fit into this concept of Sensuality. Using your imagination to become sexually aroused or think about another person is very common. Sometimes these thoughts are prompted by your senses, especially sight. Other times, fantasies might just pop into your head unprovoked. Or, you might literally dream about them while you're sleeping. Sometimes they result in a physical body response like your penis getting hard, which is called an erection. In fact, a male-bodied person may even ejaculate and have semen leave the body in their sleep, which is called a "wet dream." For more about wet dreams, check out page 66. A female-bodied person may notice that the vagina

What's porn? Porn, or pornography, can be a movie, a maga-zine or picture, or even a live web camera. People often use porn to help them fantasize about sex. Porn uses the senses of sight and sound to physically arouse people. There are lots of different kinds of porn out there for basically every kind of sexual act. There are also certain kinds of porn that are illegal (for example, porn that was not made consensually, or porn that involves minors).

Pornography is fantasy. Just like with other movies or pictures, porn is rarely real life.

Heads up: if you're under 18 and you ask for naked pictures or sexual pictures of your romantic partner, or send these types of pictures to someone, they could be considered porn. Laws vary by state. To understand how to protect yourself and your partner or friend with regard to sexting and sending or receiving pictures like this, go to: https://www.common-sensemedia.org. There is a handbook and video there that are really helpful.

If you're a teen, I suggest you stay away from taking pictures of your genitals, especially on a phone. It can get you and whomever you send it to in a lot of trouble!

Just because some people like to look at porn, it's important to remember that not everyone does. There are some people who like to incorporate porn into their sexual routines, and others who don't. Everyone is different and likes different things. Before incorporating porn into your sexual relationship, it is important for you to talk to your partner. Make sure you are both able to articulate why you want to use porn and what the expectations are for sexual behavior after you watch it.

becomes "wet" or lubricated. But that doesn't always happen. And guess what? Everyone has them. Literally *everyone*.

CIRCLE TWO: SEXUAL INTIMACY

Sexual intimacy has to do with being emotionally close to another person and accepting closeness from them. Intimacy is what makes relationships valuable. It's not just about physical intimacy, but emotional vulnerability and sharing. This emotional attachment also defines whether you "like" or "love" someone.

Caring

Intimacy with another person means that you care about them, and when you care about another person, you can empathize with them. In other words, you listen when they share their emotions and thoughts with you, and you understand where they are coming from. Likewise, in a caring, intimate relationship you can share how you're feeling with your partner—both good and bad—and feel safe doing so. You know that your partner is not going to make fun of you or belittle your feelings. Having an intimate relationship with another person is only possible when you care about the other person. If you don't care about the other person, there can't be true intimacy. Sure, you can become physically intimate with another person without caring, but that isn't true intimacy. It's a surface interaction. True intimacy will only happen when you care about your sexual partner.

Emotional Risk-Taking

Intimacy with another person depends on making yourself vulnerable while your partner does the same. True intimacy with another person will only happen when the people involved take a risk and share personal thoughts and feelings. This can be risky because you don't always know how the other person will react. Sharing your beliefs and opinions can be scary as you are opening yourself up. When you're vulnerable, you may be hurt if you're rejected, or if someone disagrees with you. There may be a time when you make yourself vulnerable, but maybe the other person isn't willing to take the same risk. Unfortunately, without really opening yourself up to another person, there is no ability to be close to another person.

CIRCLE THREE: SEXUAL IDENTITY

This circle is all about how you see yourself in the world, whether you're male or female (according to society's definitions of male and female). There are several components that make up a person's sexual identity, such as how they express their identity (otherwise known as gender role). Sometimes a person's biological sex is not the same as his or her gender identity (otherwise known as transgender). This is why I refer to people in the anatomy section as male-bodied and female-bodied. Sexual identity is such a core component of how we see ourselves operating in the world that it is extremely important to recognize and honor a person's self-identified identity.

Did you know that most children have determined their gender identity by age two?

Gender Role

A person's gender role is defined in a couple different ways. Some of the roles males and females take on are a result of their actual physical bodies, while

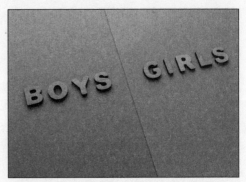

Why is blue the "boy" color? Why is pink the "girl" color? What if you don't identify as a boy or a girl? What's your color?

others are constructs of their culture. For example, only a female is physically capable of carrying a baby. Additionally, in American culture, it's not considered appropriate for a male to wear a skirt or dress. You probably hear things like, "That's a job for a man," or "That's women's work." These types of societal beliefs are changing, but they imply that our gender determines how we experience the world and whether those experiences are positive or negative depending on whether we feel aligned with our expected gender roles.

There is also a thing called "gender bias." Gender biases are stereotypical beliefs a person might hold about others based on their gender. An example of gender bias is assuming that all women are bad drivers. Or that men should not be the primary caretakers of children. People can believe these stereotypes without any supporting data just because it's what they have been taught. The more people examine these types of biases, the more cultural changes we see... but that's a whole other book!

Sexual Orientation

Whom you're attracted to sexually, your sexual orientation, is also a part of gender identity. Wait, I thought we talked about attraction in Circle One: Sensuality? We sure did! We talked about how that first circle is all about what feels good. When we talk about sexual orientation in the identity circle, we are talking more about the science of identity. Just as scientifically a person is born with certain genitalia, they are also born with a sexual orientation. A person can be heterosexual, gay, lesbian, bisexual, pansexual, or even asexual. (Sexual orientation will be explored deeper in chapter 9.) A person's sexual orientation begins to emerge during puberty as a person starts to notice whom they are attracted to.

"Recent research suggests that 11% of American adults acknowledge at least some same-sex attraction, 8.2% report that they've engaged in same-sex behavior, but only 3.5% identify as lesbian, gay, or bisexual. This shows that what people feel or do is not always the same as how they identify themselves."[5] Research also shows that people fall somewhere on the sexuality continuum and don't always fall neatly into one category or another.

Homosexual   Bisexual   Heterosexual

---

5   "What causes sexual orientation?." Planned Parenthood. Accessed January 18, 2018. https://www.plannedparenthood.org/learn/sexual-orientation-gender/sexual-orientation/what-causes-sexual-orientation.

CIRCLE FOUR: REPRODUCTION AND SEXUAL HEALTH

Aha! *Here* it is! Sex. This circle is the one you thought this book was about, but it's only one aspect of sexuality! Pretty amazing, isn't it? This circle is all about the "mechanics" of sex or the actual act of sex. This circle is all about how humans reproduce. Like, what actually happens during sexual activity. This circle also encompasses your sexual behaviors (like the sexual things you do that don't necessarily lead to the creation of another human being) and attitudes about sexual relationships (like which sexual acts you choose to do).

Reproduction and Sexual Intercourse

We will definitely be taking a deeper dive into what reproduction is in chapter 7, but basically, this is the factual and medically accurate information about how humans are made. A cell from a female-bodied person meets a cell from a male-bodied person, and, how-do-you-do, another human is formed. Knowing how that actually happens is critical to understand bodily functions and maintaining your own health (like preventing pregnancy and STIs).

Reproduction happens through sexual intercourse when using a penis and vagina. But sexual intercourse can be defined in many ways. The three main types of sexual behavior are vaginal sex (vaginal penetration either by a penis or sex toy or hand/fingers), oral sex (mouth to genitals), and anal sex (penetration of the anus with the penis or sex toy or hand/fingers). What you choose to engage in, *when you decide you're ready*, is up to you and your partner. Some people engage in all of the above, while others are only com-

40

fortable with or enjoy one type of sex. Any and all of these are okay as long as they are consensual (meaning both you and your partner are into it) and you and your partner have decided you're ready to take your relationship to the next level. There is more on consent in chapter 16 and more about figuring out if you're ready in chapter 6.

CIRCLE FIVE: SEXUALIZATION

Using sex to manipulate a situation or give yourself power over another person is called sexualization. Sexualization can be as harmless as flirting, and it also includes seduction (which means to try and make someone sexually attracted to you). It can also be cruel and lead to criminal acts like sexual harassment, abuse, and rape. No one has the right to exploit you sexually, and you don't have the right to exploit another person sexually. Please refer to chapter 16 where we discuss more about consent.

While flirting and seduction are relatively harmless, they are both forms of manipulation. Any time a person is being manipulated or using manipulation, there is a risk of one or both people being hurt or humiliated. They can also lead to sexual harassment, which means that a person is harassed because of their gender or orientation. Often, it's the recipient of the behavior that defines it as sexual harassment. For example, at school you might be patted on the butt by a schoolmate. The person who touched your butt might think they were flirting, but you feel intimidated and violated. If you feel this way, you may call it sexual harassment. Sexual harassment can range from inappropriate comments to inappropriate or unwanted touches (anywhere on the body). Sexual harassment is illegal and you have the right to file a complaint against another person who you perceive to be sexually harassing you. Similarly, if another person feels harassed by you, they have the right to file a complaint against you.

Rape and incest are two behaviors that are illegal and fit into this circle of sexualization. Rape happens when you coerce or are coerced into having genital contact with another person. Rape can happen to anyone and it can be by someone you know. It isn't always like what you see on TV. Incest is a type of rape or forced sexual contact on a minor by someone who is related to them. Sexual assault, of any kind, is never okay. Please refer to chapter 18 where we discuss consent, a person's rights, and resources for victims.

CONVERSATION STARTERS . . .
• • • • • • • • • •

The conversation starters are designed to be prompts for having conversations. Feel free to use them in the way that feels right to you.

Questions for Teens to Ask Their Parents:

- What parts of the circles seemed familiar to you? Was there anything that was surprising? Which parts? Why?

- Based on what you learned when you looked at the circles of sexuality, has your perception of anything changed? If yes, what?

- The messages I've gotten about Sensuality/Sexual Intimacy/Gender Identity/Reproduction/Sexualization are_____.

- Growing up, did you ever experience a negative situation or hear negative messages that you didn't agree with? What are some positive messages that you got growing up?

Questions for Parents to Ask Their Teens:

- What messages (from your family, from the media, from friends) have you gotten about Sensuality? Sexual Intimacy? Gender Identity? Reproduction? Sexualization?

- Where have these messages come from? Do you feel like they are reinforced or different in your family? What about school? What messages do you get from

43

your friends or partner? (Discuss differences if there are any and what might cause them.)

- Do you think it's important to talk about different aspects of the circles with a romantic partner? What parts? Why? (If your teen has not identified parts you would hope they talk to their partner about, mention those and explain why.)

6

HOW DO YOU KNOW
WHEN YOU'RE READY?

THINGS TO THINK ABOUT WHEN DECIDING TO BECOME SEXUALLY ACTIVE

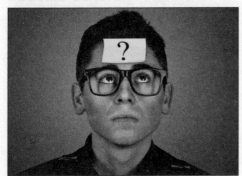

Everyone struggles with the question, "When is the right time to have sex?" Literally, everyone.

There is no exactly "right" time to become sexually active. I can't tell you that. For every person, it's different. Which is how it should be because we all experience life in different ways, are involved in different relationships, and have different values. According to research, people become sexually active around the age of seventeen.[6] That's

---

6   Finer LB and Philbin JM, *Trends in ages at key reproductive transitions in the United States*, 1951–2010, Women's Health Issues, 2014, 24(3): e271-e279.

the average. So, for some it's earlier and for some it's later. Only you get to decide when you want to have sex. And there are going to be a lot of different messages coming at you, all trying to tell you one thing or another. You will hear advice at school, you might see things on TV or in a movie, your parents or other family members might be giving you different messages. You need to stay true to you. What's your value? Because only you know when it's right for you.

I want to be sure to mention that some people do not have a choice about when they first have sex because they have survived sexual assault. Meaning, they were forced to have sex. Their choice was taken from them, and that is not okay. If you have experienced sexual assault and have not already told someone, can you? Is there someone that it's safe to tell? If you can't identify someone, you can call 800-656-HOPE (4673) or go to www.rainn.org. It could be helpful for you to get some support. Your history does not dictate how or when you have sex in the future.

So, how do you figure out when it's the "right" time for you? Reading this book is a great place to start. It's important to have as much information about what sex is and what the risks are before you have sex. Talking to your parents (or another adult you trust) is also a really great thing to do. As hard as it might be to believe it, your parents have actually been in the same place, wondering when they should have sex for the first time. It doesn't mean you have to do the same thing that they did, because every person's experience is vastly different. But talking through a big step like this with someone you trust can help you to see all the sides of the issue and make a really informed decision.

Other things you will want to consider are your belief systems and values. Thinking about all the risks involved in being sexually active is important. Understanding how sex has the potential to impact your life is major. If you value education and graduating high school, how might sexual activity impact that? Are you religious? If so, what does your religion say about sex? You get to determine which values you want to ascribe to. Ideally, being sexually active is not something you're ashamed of or feel bad about.

Consider whether you have access to a health care provider. If you're at risk for becoming pregnant once you become sexually active, are you on contraception? Once you become sexually active, regardless of the kind of sex you have, how will you make sure you and your partner are healthy (as in you have the ability to get tested and possibly treated for Sexually Transmitted Infections, or STIs). If you're female-bodied, do you have irregular periods? We look deeper at STIs in chapter 13 and at contraception in chapter 14.

What about your partner? Have you talked about being sexually active? What's your relationship like? Do you trust your partner and feel safe with them? Have you discussed what your sexual boundaries are? This isn't a one-way street, and sex doesn't "just happen." There are actually a number of things you and your partner should talk about before getting it on. This book goes pretty in-depth about setting up boundaries, communication, healthy relationships, and consent. Check out chapters 16 and 17.

In order to know if you're ready for sexual activity, I suggest taking a deep look at your life, your goals, and your relationship, and making sure you understand how being sexually active may impact your life. Below are some questions you can ask yourself and your partner. How you answer the questions might give you a better idea of whether you're ready or not. Remember: sexuality is a lifetime thing, so you've got lots of time to have sex. Regardless of what you might hear from friends or media, there is no perfect age or time or situation to become sexually active. Also, answering the questions isn't going to give you some magical calendar date. It isn't a prediction of your behavior. Circumstances change, relationships change. These questions are only out there to help get you thinking about when you might think it's time.

I also want to make sure that if you have already had sex, and maybe you weren't sure you should have had sex, you can stop. Even if you're already sexually active, I think going through the questions can help you figure out if you want to keep having sex or if you want to engage in different behaviors. Having sex or engaging in sexual activity of some kind doesn't mean you're resigned to always engage in that activity. For sure check out chapter 16 for more on consent.

Being sexually active is not about anyone but you. Here are some questions to think about when you're trying to decide whether you're ready for sex: [7]

- Is your decision to have sex completely your own (you feel no pressure from others, including your partner)?

- Is your decision to have sex based on the right

---

7   Posted under Health Guides. Updated 17 May 2017. Related Content. "Making Healthy Sexual Decisions." Center for Young Women's Health. Accessed January 17, 2018. https://youngwomenshealth.org/2013/05/23/making-healthy-sexual-decisions/.

reasons? (It shouldn't be based on peer pressure, a need to fit in or make your partner happy, or a belief that sex is the only way to make your relationship with your partner better, or closer. If you decide to have sex, it should be because you feel emotionally and physically ready. Your partner should be someone you trust.)

- Do you feel your partner would respect any decision you made about whether to have sex or not?

- Are you able to comfortably talk to your partner about sex and your partner's sexual history?

- Have you and your partner talked about what both of you would do if you became pregnant or got an STI?

- Do you know how to prevent pregnancy and STIs?

- Are you and your partner willing to use contraception to prevent pregnancy and STIs?

- Do you really feel ready and completely comfortable with yourself and your partner to have sex?

There's no magical age to start having sex. But, I can tell you, you probably are *not* ready if the reasons you have for considering having sex include anything like:

- I don't want to be the only person in my group of friends who isn't having sex

- I just don't want to be a virgin anymore

- I will have more friends if I have sex

- People will see me as more mature if I am having sex

WHAT DOES IT MEAN TO "FEEL HORNY?"

One reason people have sex is because they feel "horny." But what does that even mean? And if you feel horny, does that mean you are ready to have sex?

If someone "feels horny," it means they feel sexually aroused. Maybe they are watching something or see a picture of something and they feel their body responding sexually, or their thoughts become sexual. Some people become sexually aroused by listening to certain sounds. Every person is different. As a person is exposed to more things, what arouses them may change. Everybody experiences arousal differently. Feeling horny can be both a mental and physical experience, or just one or the other. For some people, it's more physical and for others, it's more mental. Some reactions include an erection (for a male-bodied person), increased vaginal discharge (for a female-bodied person), increased heartrate, increased sweating, or having a hard time concentrating. Basically, a person can become sexually aroused, or "horny," as a result of having any of their senses stimulated. And what makes one person feel horny doesn't always do it for another person.

A person who is horny may or may not be ready for sex. Just because something is "making you feel horny" does not mean that you need to have sex. If that were true, there are some people who would be having sex, like, all the time. A person's gotta sleep, amiright? Feeling horny is just an indication that something or someone is arousing.

It's true that some people feel so horny (or so aroused) that they feel some sort of release is important. Again, this doesn't necessarily mean that you need to engage in sex. Masturbation is a way of satisfying yourself without having sex and is a great option for those who don't know if

MAKING SENSE OF "IT"

they are ready for sex. For more on what masturbation is, go to chapter 11. But many people don't need to have sex or masturbate when they feel horny because the urges and sensations you feel can go away with time. If you don't have sex or masturbate when you feel horny, you will be perfectly okay. This will not hurt your body. You need to do what feels right for you.

CONVERSATION STARTERS . . .

. . . .

The conversation starters are designed to be prompts for having conversations. Feel free to use them in the way that feels right to you.

Questions for Teens to Ask Their Parents

- How did you know when you were ready to have sex for the first time?

- Do you wish you could change anything about the first time you had sex?

Questions for Parents to Ask Their Teens

- What sorts of things do you want in a relationship before becoming sexually active with a partner?

- Do you ever feel pressure to be sexually active? From whom? How can I support you?

7

OUR BODIES ARE PRETTY AMAZING (AND DO SOME CRAZY STUFF)

REPRODUCTIVE BIOLOGY, PUBERTY, SEXUAL ACTIVITY, MASTURBATION, AND MORE!

In order to be able to talk about sex, it's going to be important to understand what bodies look like and what they can do. Whether you're male-bodied or female-bodied, it's good to have a general understanding of the different parts and what they do. This understanding can also help you advocate for yourself with your doctor (if something isn't feeling right) and help you talk to your partner when telling them what you do and do not want to do sexually. Our bodies are pretty amazing and do some crazy stuff, so it's important to understand the biology of pregnancy as well as parenting options and support.

When it comes to the reproductive anatomy, some people like to use slang terms. It's okay if you want to use these slang terms because you might be more comfortable doing that, but if you use slang terms, your partner or doctor might not know what you're talking about. So, for the purposes of learning, we are going to use the medical terminology for the reproductive parts. You can refer to the drawing of the reproductive parts on pages 55, 58, 61, 71, 75, and 76 as we talk about the different parts and what they do. In order to do this, we are going to look at some diagrams that show what male-bodied and female-bodied people look like after they have gone through puberty. The drawings have labels so you know the names of all the different parts. What those parts do comes in the rest of the pages in this chapter.

Wait, I don't look like those drawings!

The drawings used are to give you a general idea of what the genitalia look like. Your genitalia, most likely, looks different. Everybody's does. Use what you see to get a general idea of what some male-bodied person and female-bodied person's genitalia look like.

I've Got Some Questions...

"You keep using these terms 'male-bodied' and 'female-bodied.' I don't understand why..." Basically, a person may have been born with male genitalia and not identify as a male. Same goes for a person born with female genitalia. Using the terms "male-bodied" and "female-bodied" aims to be more inclusive. Please take a look at the information in Chapter 9 for a deeper dive into this topic area.

MALE ANATOMY

Let's start with a male body. There are parts on the outside and parts on the inside that make up the male anatomy. Every male-bodied person's penis and scrotum look different. If we look inside, we will see all the parts that make hormones and semen. On the outside, we can see the scrotum and penis.

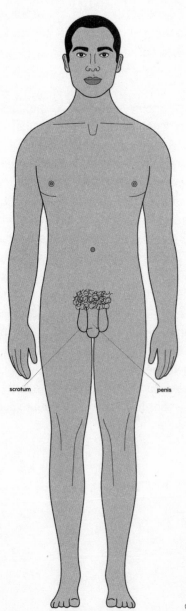

scrotum

penis

©2017 Sofie Birkin

Alrighty, now we know the names, but what do they *do*? Let's start with the part you probably already knew about (at least, what it was called).

Penis

The penis is commonly referred to as the male sex organ. It can be used to penetrate the vagina or anus. The urethra, or the tube that the urine or pee comes out of, is also in the penis. Urine comes out of a small hole at the tip of the penis. This is also where a male-bodied person's pre-ejaculate (or "pre-cum") and ejaculate (or "cum," the fluid that contains sperm) leaves the body. The penis is actually two parts: the **shaft** and the **glans**. The **shaft** is usually what we think of when we talk about the penis. It's the long, tube-like part of the penis. This part of the penis is made of a soft sponge-like material on the inside. This material can fill with blood, making the penis erect, or hard. When the penis becomes erect, it grows in length and width. A penis usually becomes erect when a male-bodied person becomes sexually aroused. But it can also become hard spontaneously. Check out more on this on page 66. The shaft of the penis (whether hard or soft) is very sensitive to touch because there are a lot of nerves in the penis.

> **FUN FACT:** Did you know that a male cannot ejaculate if the penis isn't hard?
>
> **FUN FACT:** A penis can become erect for other reasons besides being sexually aroused. This kind of erection, called a "spontaneous erection," can happen without being sexually aroused and is fairly common, especially when a male-bodied person goes through puberty.
>
> **FUN FACT:** When the penis is soft, or flaccid, it typically measures 1-3 inches in length. If it becomes erect, or hard, it will grow to be 4-6 inches long on average.

The other part of the penis is called the **glans**. This is the tip of the penis and it's super sensitive. The glans of the penis on a male-bodied person is relative to the clitoris on the female-bodied person. There is a bundle of nerves there that, when stimulated, can lead to orgasm. (Check out more about having an orgasm on page 120.)

The **glans** may or may not have skin covering it. This skin is called **foreskin**, which is attached to the **glans** with a piece of skin called the **frenulum**. If there is not skin over the glans, the penis is considered *circumcised*. (Typically, even if the male-bodied person has been circumcised there is some portion of the **frenulum** remaining). If there is skin present, the penis is called *uncircumcised*. The decision on whether a male-bodied person is circumcised or not can depend on culture, religion and parental preference.

FUN FACT: Today, a little more than half of male-bodied individuals in the U.S. are circumcised shortly after they are born. Circumcision may be more common in certain areas of the country than in others, or in certain cultures and religions.[8]

On the left you can see a drawing of what a circumcised penis looks like, and on the right is a drawing of an uncircumcised penis.[9]

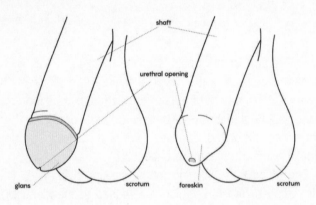

Circumcised penis   **Unircumcised penis**

©2017 Sofie Birkin

The picture on the left is a drawing of what a circumcised penis looks like. The drawing on the right is a picture of an uncircumcised penis. The uncircumcised penis looks like the circumcised penis when the skin surrounding the head of the penis (the foreskin) is pushed back.

---

8 Team, The BabyCenter Editorial. "How many baby boys get circumcised?" BabyCenter. September 27, 2015. Accessed January 17, 2018. http://www.babycenter.com/404_how-many-baby-boys-get-circumcised_10331716.bc.

9 "Are My Penis & Testicles Normal? | Facts About Male Anatomy." Planned Parenthood. Accessed January 17, 2018. http://www.plannedparenthood.org/learn/teens/puberty/are-my-penis-and-testicles-normal

Whether circumcised or not, penises work the same way—they just look a little different and can feel a little different to the person with whom the male-bodied person is having sex. Self-care is also going to look slightly different. For example, if a male-bodied person is uncircumcised, they may need to pull the foreskin back when they urinate and wash their genitals. If they use a condom during sex, that also might look a little different. We will go into that more when we talk about condom use in chapter 14.

All penises look a little different from each other. And we aren't just referring to whether or not they are circumcised. Some penises curve a little (in any direction) when erect. Some penises are darker in color than the rest of the male's body. Penises can be long when they are flaccid and only grow a little bit when erect; they can be small when flaccid and grow a lot when erect; or they can be small when flaccid and not grow a lot when erect. Every penis is different, and there is no "perfect" penis. A lot of male-bodied people are worried about the shape and size of their penis and what their partner thinks about their penis. Just remember, it isn't the penis shape or size that matters, it is how a male-bodied person treats their partner during sexual activity that leads to pleasure.

Scrotum
The scrotum is responsible for holding the testicles. The scrotum is covered with wrinkled skin and sometimes pubic hair. The scrotum's job is to protect the testicles by bringing the testicles closer to the body if it is too cold or by loosening the hold on the testicles to move them further away from the body if the body is too hot. This job is important because the testicles need to be at the exact right

temperature in order to make sperm. Just like the penis, no scrotum looks like another scrotum. They can be big or small, have a little or a lot of hair, and vary in color.

If we were able to look through the skin of the scrotum, we would see the testicles. Some people call the testicles "nuts" or "balls," among other things. Most male-bodied people are born with two testicles. No matter how many testicles a person has, though, they all produce the same two main things: sperm and a hormone called *testosterone*. We'll get into the amazing world of testicles when we look inside the male-bodied person's body.

The last part of the male body that I'll mention doesn't specifically belong to the reproductive anatomy, but is still important because it can be involved in sexual activity. I'm referring to the anal opening. The anal opening can be a source of sexual pleasure. The anal opening is located between the butt cheeks, and the anus is where solid waste, or poop/feces, leaves the body. During sexual activity, a finger, sex toy, or penis may be inserted into the anus (either along the opening of the anus—the rectum—or inside the anus). This is called *anal sex*.

LOOKING ON THE INSIDE

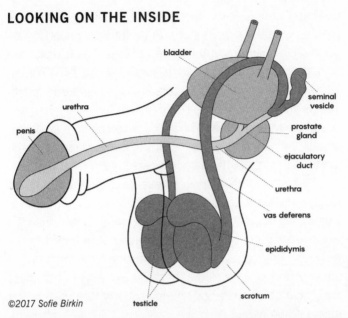

This illustration gives you a good overview of all the tubes and glands that make up the male reproductive system. Despite a fairly simple exterior, the male-bodied reproductive system is quite complex.

Urethra

We've already reviewed the long tube that is inside the penis: the urethra. As a reminder, this is the tube through which urine (from the bladder), semen, and pre-ejaculate exit the body. When you're looking at the picture, be sure to note that the urethra is attached to the bladder and the testicles (by way of a lot of other organs).

Testicles

The testicles are two ball-like glands inside the scrotum that produce the sperm and testosterone. Testicles are always making sperm. At least, they are always making sperm once the male-bodied person starts to go through puberty. Testicles are a sperm factory that never stops. The testicles are on duty, creating millions and millions of sperm 24/7/365. In other words, a male-bodied person will never stop producing sperm for as long as they live (unless they have their testicles removed). As a male-bodied person ages, their sperm production may slow down, but it will keep on keepin' on no matter how old the male-bodied person is.

Most male-bodied people have two testicles that are roughly the same size. But a lot of people have one that is bigger than the other or one that hangs a little lower than the other—totally normal. Testosterone is also produced in the testicles. This hormone starts production in earnest during puberty and is responsible for the many physical changes that occur to the male body during puberty (see page 65 for more info on puberty).

Testicles are also pretty sensitive when they are touched (through the thin skin of the scrotum). If they are hit or twisted, it can be extremely painful. (A common misconception is that the scrotum is what is sensitive, but, as we now know, the scrotum is just a thin layer of skin—a testicle purse, if you will.) Any male-bodied person should always protect their testicles when they play sports by wearing a cup and compression underwear. Since the testicles are so sensitive, this means that it can be pleasurable for a male-bodied person to have their testicles gently massaged, rubbed, or stroked. As with any sexual activity, check with your partner about what they like and don't like. Just because it can be sexually stimulating doesn't mean that you or your partner like them to be touched.

Sperm

The **sperm** is a type of cell (only visible by microscope) that is responsible for helping to create a human if it meets with an egg from a female-bodied person. When viewed under a microscope it looks like this:

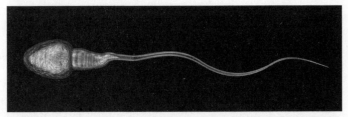

Here's a photo of what an actual sperm looks like under a microscope. It only takes one sperm to meet an egg to form a baby. The head on the sperm is the part that contains the DNA and all the good stuff needed to make a baby. The long tail is just the way it gets places. Once the sperm meets the egg, the tail actually comes off.

You can't see sperm unless it's under a microscope. So, when a male-bodied person ejaculates, the fluid that comes out contains millions and millions of sperm combined with other fluid. Sperm need that fluid to survive. It contains food and nutrients that keep the sperm alive and wiggly. The wiggliness of the sperm is really important. It's caused by the tail of the sperm. That tail propels the sperm and gets them where they are supposed to go, which, according to biology, is towards the egg (provided by a female-bodied person). If the sperm were to meet an egg, the head of the sperm—the part that contains DNA—would enter the egg and together they would grow to form a human embryo. Although a male-bodied person ejaculates millions and millions of sperm, it only takes one of those to meet the egg and form a pregnancy.

Hold up, what's DNA? That's short for deoxyribonucleic acid, the molecule that contains the genetic code and what makes you, you! And, if you decided to have a child using this sperm, that child would have some of the same characteristics based on that DNA.

As we already mentioned, sperm aren't made in the male body until that person goes through puberty. Once a male-bodied person goes through puberty, they are always making sperm. Just because the body is always making it, though, doesn't mean it has to be used. Luckily, the human body is pretty amazing and, since the sperm are so tiny, the testicles can also store the sperm until they are needed (as in ejaculated), like a built-in warehouse. Even though the testicles are storing sperm, they will not get larger because they are storing the sperm. So there isn't any need to be worried that they are going to become too full or overflow—it's impossible. I told you, human bodies are pretty amazing!

FUN FACT: While it might seem like a lot, the male-bodied person only ejaculates a little more than half a teaspoon of semen! The majority of the fluid is actually made up of water. One reason it may seem like more is because it leaves the body so fast and can actually go a long way. An average male-bodied person ejaculates at a speed of 28 miles per hour, and the world record for how far a male-bodied person has ejaculated is 18 feet, 9 inches!

Each ejaculation contains an average of 200 million sperm, while pre-ejaculate can have up to 40 million sperm in it![10]

What's puberty for a male-bodied person?

Okay, hold it, now. What the heck is puberty, you ask? Well, it's the time in a person's life when they go through physical and emotional developmental changes. For male-bodied people, puberty typically starts between twelve and sixteen. But that doesn't mean it can't start earlier or later. The start of puberty is triggered by the pituitary gland in the brain. This part of the brain talks to the testicles and tells them to start making the testosterone hormone. This hormone is responsible for different physical changes like making a person's voice deeper, and growing hair on the genitals, in the armpits, on the chest, and on the face. It's also responsible for increasing the breadth of a male-bodied person's shoulders. Other changes in puberty include the face starting

---

10 "10 Things You Didn't Know about Your Orgasms." Men's Health. June 06, 2017. Accessed January 17, 2018. http://www.menshealth.com/sex-women/10-things-about-orgasms.

News, CBS. "Sperm: 15 crazy things you should know." CBS News. September 19, 2011. Accessed January 17, 2018. http://www.cbsnews.com/pictures/sperm-15-crazy-things-you-should-know/12/.

to create more oil (leading to increased acne) and major growing spurts. Not only will a male-bodied person grow in height, but they will notice that the penis will begin to grow, too.

Additionally, a male-bodied person may have spontaneous erections (the penis becomes hard as it fills with blood, typically without feeling sexually aroused). These erections can happen when you're sitting in math class trying to figure out a math problem, they can happen when you're watching a movie, and they can happen when you're sleeping. Basically, they can happen at any time, anywhere—thus the "spontaneous" part of the name. A male-bodied person in puberty will also start to have nocturnal emissions (which is the technical term for "wet dreams").

Wet dreams are when a male-bodied person releases semen (don't worry, I'll get into what semen is in a minute) while they are sleeping, usually without even knowing it until the person wakes up. Most male-bodied people have wet dreams occasionally, but as they get older, they won't have them as often. Also, a male-bodied person's penis can become hard while they sleep without ejaculating. A lot of male-bodied people observe this by having an erection when they wake up. The slang term for this is "morning wood." (BTW, a female-bodied person can also have a wet dream. For female-bodied people this is usually less physically noticeable because the fluid usually stays inside the body.)

Puberty is also when a male-bodied person typically begins to have sexual feelings. Sexual feelings include not only being attracted to someone physically (as in, thinking another person is "cute"), but wanting to act on those feelings of attraction. There is a desire to be sexual, even just kiss and hold hands, with a person that might not have been there before. Seeing, thinking about, or touching the person can lead to a heightened sense of sexual arousal that may or may not lead to an erection. This is sometimes called being "horny." I went into more on what "being horny" is on page 50, but basically, it's feeling sexually aroused to the point you want to engage in sexual activity (either with the person or through masturbation and touching your genitals).

Because puberty is the first time these feelings become really strong, this is around the time that a person starts to understand their sexual orientation (who they are attracted to). They might find they are attracted to a different gender (heterosexual) or the same gender (homosexual). For some people this is really clear and they can see themselves clearly as orienting towards a certain gender. For others, determining who they are attracted to isn't as clear. In fact, a lot of people go throughout their teen years feeling attracted to lots of different kinds of people and various genders. For more on sexual orientation, go to chapter 9. The teen years are very complicated and this concept of sexual attraction doesn't make it any easier. Be patient with yourself. You will figure it out. Just make sure you have someone to talk to (like your parents and/or a good friend who you can trust). And make sure you're safe! If you're going to try to engage in sexual acts with anyone, regardless of gender, make sure you know how to keep yourself safe from STIs, pregnancy, and risky situations.

Back to the rest of the male reproductive anatomy and the journey of the sperm . . .
Once the sperm (or I should say, millions of sperm) are created inside the testicle, they travel into what is called the **epididymis**. This is basically where the sperm go to "grow

up" and learn how to do what they were created to do (meet the egg). Growing up means they're fully developing, practicing their swimming, you know, practicing for their big debut. The epididymis is a tube that is tightly coiled up on top of, and behind, each testicle. Like the testicles, sperm like to hang out here, too. The epididymis will also act like a storage tank for sperm until the body needs them. Again, the epididymis won't become too full and get bigger with more and more sperm.

Each epididymis has a long narrow tube attached to it called a **vas deferens**. The job of the vas deferens is to carry the sperm from the epididymis to the seminal vesicles during ejaculation. **Seminal vesicles** are two small organs that produce what is called "seminal fluid." This fluid provides proteins that keep the sperm alive as they continue along their journey out of the body.

After visiting the seminal vesicle, the sperm journey to the **prostate gland**. The prostate adds more fluid, which helps reduce friction as the sperm leave the body and gives the sperm what they need to finish their journey (food, camping gear, emergency flashlights—j/k!). Nutrients. Just boring nutrients. The prostate gland is about the size of a golf ball and is really sensitive to pressure. It can be felt through the anal opening and, as a male-bodied person gets older, doctors check the health of the prostate by inserting their fingers into the rectum (the opening of the anus) and pressing on the prostate while the male coughs. The prostate is sometimes called the male-bodied person's "G-spot." For more on what the G-spot is, go to page 80. Once the sperm have gone through the prostate gland, we can call the fluid **semen**.

Now that the male body has produced semen, it's ready

to leave the body. Semen will only leave the body when the male-bodied individual is physically ready to release the semen. In other words, the male-bodied person is sexually aroused and getting ready to ejaculate. (The semen is produced regardless of why the male-bodied person is ejaculating—if they are having penis-to-vagina sex, masturbating, or having a wet dream, all of these situations can end in a male-bodied person ejaculating semen).

However, before the male-bodied person ejaculates out the urethra, something really important needs to happen: the urethra needs to be cleaned out so that the semen can safely leave the body. And by safely leave the body, I mean that the sperm remain viable or alive and ready to do what they are biologically designed to do: find an egg. (Spoiler alert: a sperm doesn't know what it is leaving the body to do; it just knows it has been set free and goes on autopilot.) This means that the sperm within the semen are given the best possible chance of surviving.

Because the urethra serves a dual purpose for a male-bodied person (remember, it's the tube that urine, or pee, uses to exit the body), the body will produce what is called **pre-ejaculate**, or pre-cum, to clean out the urethra. This pre-ejaculate fluid does not mix with the semen; rather, it comes out right before a male-bodied person ejaculates. It makes sure that any urine, which can make the urethra a hostile environment for sperm to survive, is cleaned out. In addition to cleaning the urethra out, it provides more lubrication so that the semen has an easier time leaving the body.

Pre-ejaculate is made in the **Cowper's Gland**. That's the Cowper's Gland's only job—to create the cleaning fluid for the urethra. While pre-ejaculate comes from a separate gland than semen, it's important to remember that it's

69

possible for pre-ejaculate fluid to contain sperm. This means that if the pre-ejaculate comes into contact with a female-bodied person's vaginal opening, that female-bodied person runs a higher risk of becoming pregnant. Even if there isn't sperm present in the pre-ejaculate, if the male-bodied person has an STI, the pre-ejaculate can also carry that STI. Therefore, any person who comes in contact with the pre-ejaculate runs the risk of contracting an STI. When we talk about how to protect you or a partner from STIs and/or pregnancy in chapter 13 and chapter 14, it is important to remember that a condom, for example, would need to go on the penis before the pre-ejaculate leaves the body in order to mitigate the risk of transmission and/or pregnancy.

FEMALE ANATOMY

Now that we have a general understanding of what the male reproductive anatomy does and what it looks like, it's time to become more familiar with what a female-bodied person's reproductive organs are and what they do. What are the parts found outside the female body?

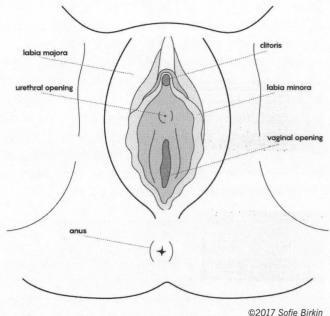

labia majora

clitoris

urethral opening

labia minora

vaginal opening

anus

©2017 Sofie Birkin

In this illustration you can see that the openings to the vagina, urethra and anus are very different. Of course every female-bodied person's vulva looks different.

When we look at the whole area between a female-bodied person's legs, this is called the **vulva**. The vulva includes the clitoris, labia, and opening to the vagina. This area is also referred to as the genitals. And a lot of people generally refer to this whole area as the vagina (although that is actually not medically accurate). In order to understand the female body's genitals, or the parts of the vulva, let's start at the top, at the clitoris. The **clitoris** is actually bigger than what you can see or feel on the outside of the body. It's kind of like an iceberg—there is a small amount of skin on the out-side, but internally, the clitoris extends down on both sides through the labia and around the vaginal wall.

Every female-bodied person's clitoris looks different. Some people have larger (fatter and/or longer) clitorises, while others' clitorises are smaller. The clitoris's only purpose is pleasure. That's it. It's extremely sensitive as it is made up of nerves (similar to the glans on the penis). Stimulation of the clitoris can be pleasurable for female-bodied people, and many female-bodied people use the clitoris during both sexual intercourse and masturbation.

> **FUN FACT:** Many female-bodied people can only achieve orgasm when their clitoris is stimulated. This is why many sex toys are smaller vibrators intended to remain outside the body; they are specifically designed for clitoral stimulation.

While the clitoris is the "exciting" and pleasurable part of the woman's external reproductive anatomy, the other parts are equally important to know. So, as you look down from the clitoris, you will see the **urethral opening**. The urethral opening is where pee or urine comes out. That's it. Nothing else should be coming out of this opening and nothing can go inside it. While technically not a part of the reproductive anatomy, the urethra is right there with all the other parts, so you need to know that this is where the pee comes out. (Note, a lot of people get confused and think the pee comes out of the vagina because they are so close together. Also, some female-bodied people, upon orgasming, have a lot of vaginal discharge leave their body. That does come out of the vagina.) If there is something else coming out of the urethral opening besides pee, then you (and maybe your partner, depending on your diagnosis) should go to a health care provider and get it checked out.

The urethral opening is really small, and besides maybe a medical instrument, you aren't going to be able to put anything inside the urethra. A lot of female-bodied people are nervous that a finger, tampon, sex toy, or penis might get inserted in there because it gets confused with the vaginal opening. But don't worry! Nothing can get inserted in there.

The place where things can get inserted is the **vaginal opening** (which is right below the urethra). So, this is where you would put a tampon during a period (if you choose to use tampons), or where a penis, sex toy, or finger might go in during sexual activity. This is also where some forms of contraception are inserted. The vagina is also the opening where a baby would come out.

The clitoris, urethral opening, and vaginal opening are all covered by skin called **labia**. There is a set of labia on each female-bodied person. There are actually two sets of labia: the **inner labia** and the **outer labia**. While there are two sets, their function is very much the same. These flaps of skin serve as protection for the vaginal opening, clitoris and urethral opening. The labia usually change color (becoming darker) and get bigger during puberty (for more information on puberty, head to page 80.) They also swell with blood when a female-bodied person becomes sexually aroused. They don't get hard like a penis does, but they become more sensitive to touch.

The last two parts of the female body that don't specifically belong to the reproductive anatomy, but are important to note because they are often used during sexual activity, are the anal opening and the breasts. These can both be used as a source of sexual pleasure. The anal opening is located a little farther below the vaginal opening. The anus is where solid waste, or poop/feces, leaves the body. During sexual activity, a finger, sex toy or penis may be inserted into the anus (either along the opening of the anus—the rectum—or inside the anus). This is called *anal sex*.

The breasts on a female-bodied person exist to produce milk during and after a pregnancy. They are extremely sensitive and can also be stimulated to create pleasure during sexual activity. Everybody's breasts look different. Some are big, some are small, and most female-bodied people have one breast that is slightly bigger than the other breast. As a female-bodied person goes through puberty, not only do the breasts grow, but nipples can also change color and grow bigger. Some people also grow hair around their nipples during puberty.

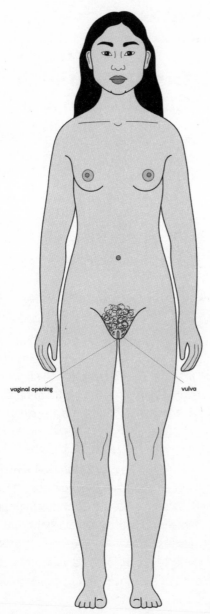

vaginal opening

vulva

©2017 Sofie Birkin

Now let's take a look inside...

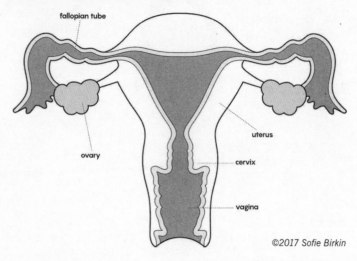

©2017 Sofie Birkin

This disembodied drawing can help you understand the relationship of the various female-bodied internal reproductive organs.

The inside of the female body is where the majority of the reproductive organs are. As we are learning about the different parts, we are also going to get a better understanding of the menstrual cycle (otherwise known as a period).

Ovaries

The **ovaries** are where the eggs are stored. A female-bodied person is born with all the eggs they will ever have. Unlike the male-bodied person who starts producing sperm during puberty, a female-bodied person is born with millions of eggs in her ovaries. However, she doesn't start releasing them until puberty. Each egg is smaller than a grain of sand, invisible to the naked eye, and can only be seen with a microscope.

Most female-bodied people are born with two ovaries. In addition to storing the eggs, or ovum, the ovaries produce the sex hormones estrogen and progesterone. These hormones are responsible for a wide range of changes that occur in the female body during puberty such as the development of breasts, hips widening, and the start of a period (which means the female-bodied person is capable of reproducing). These changes can happen fairly quickly or take several years. Everybody is different.

Once a female-bodied person starts menstruating, her ovaries will take turns releasing one egg. This process is called **ovulation** and usually happens once a month. It's possible for a woman to release more than one egg at a time, but this is not very common. If a woman does release multiple eggs during ovulation, and those eggs become fertilized with sperm, she could become pregnant with multiple embryos. An **embryo** is what the clump of fertilized cells is called before it develops into what is called a **fetus**. And the fetus is what a baby is called prior to viability. In other words, a fetus cannot live outside the uterus. But we are getting ahead of ourselves.

Fallopian Tubes

Once the ovaries release the egg, the **fallopian tubes** start their job. The fallopian tubes are about the width of uncooked spaghetti. At the end of the fallopian tubes near the ovaries are what are called **fimbriae**. The fimbriae are finger-like projections that grab the egg once it's released from the ovary. The egg then travels down one of the tubes (whichever tube is next to the ovary it was released from). This journey can take a few days and ends with the egg going into the uterus.

If a female-bodied person has sex with a male-bodied person and an **egg** has been released and is in the fallopian tube, a female-bodied person is at risk for becoming pregnant. This is most commonly when fertilization happens. Or, in other words, when a sperm meets an egg. The next stop for either the egg or **embryo** (fertilized egg) is the uterus.

Uterus

The **uterus** is a strong muscle about the size of a closed fist. Its role in reproduction is to grow the fertilized egg into a baby. The uterus, over the course of the menstrual cycle, grows a thick, nutrient-rich lining. This lining is full of blood and an ideal place for an egg to live and grow, *if* it has been fertilized by a sperm. If the egg has not been fertilized, the uterus will begin to shed its lining. This blood then exits the body and is called **menstrual blood** or a **period**. If the egg has been fertilized, it will implant into the uterine wall and develop into a fetus. This is where a baby will grow for approximately 40 weeks.

It's possible for the fertilized egg to implant in the fallopian tube. This is called an ectopic pregnancy. It is really rare but extremely unsafe for the female-bodied person. Because it's so dangerous, it must be terminated for the health of the female-bodied person.

Cervix

The **cervix** serves as a gatekeeper for the body. Although it's a gatekeeper, it does have a very small opening. This opening is super small and only big enough to let sperm in or period blood out. Basically, it keeps whatever is supposed to stay inside the uterus, inside the uterus. So, if a female-bodied person becomes pregnant, the cervix is responsible for ensuring the uterus keeps the pregnancy in the uterus until the body is ready to give birth. When a female-bodied person is ready to give birth, the cervix dilates, or opens up, wide enough for the baby to be born.

Similarly, the cervix keeps things that aren't supposed to go into the uterus out of the uterus. For example, if a penis enters the vagina, it can't go into the uterus. Also, if a female-bodied person uses a tampon for her menstrual flow, the tampon can't "get lost" inside the body because the cervix makes sure it doesn't.

Vagina

Like the uterus, the **vagina** is also a muscle and it measures, on average, 3-5 inches deep. As we mentioned already, this is where a penis would go if that's the type of sex you're engaging in. It's also where a tampon might go if you choose to use a tampon. Since it's a muscle, it can stretch to fit what goes inside (width-wise, not lengthwise). So, if a penis is wide, the vagina will stretch to fit its width. After sexual activity, the vagina will resume its normal size. Even after a baby passes through the vagina, it will return to how it was after time.

Inside the vagina is something called a **hymen**. The hymen is a thin membrane that stretches across the vaginal opening. Most female-bodied people are born with them, but everybody is different and some people aren't born with them. The membrane is typically tightly stretched across the vagina (inside the vagina) and has a small opening in it. Every person's hymen is a little different, and it's possible for some people to have two holes in the hymen. The hole is present to allow menstrual blood to flow through it. If a female-bodied person chooses to use a tampon, it can also go through the opening and, contrary to a common myth out there, a tampon *cannot* put a hole in the hymen. It might stretch the hole. And, in fact, when a female-bodied person first has vaginal sex with a penis or penis-like sex toy, it's the further stretching of the hymen that can cause some discomfort and a small amount of blood to be present. Unlike the vagina, the hymen is not a muscle designed to expand and contract. In some female-bodied people it is thicker and in some it is thinner, but once it is stretched out, it will remain stretched out.

What's a G-spot? The "G-spot" is typically associated with a female-bodied person. It's called "G-spot" after the person who "discovered" it, Ernst Gräfenberg. He was a gynecologist who discovered that some female-bodied people have an extremely sensitive area inside their vagina that, when stimulated, can lead to orgasm and female ejaculation. The G-spot is a little controversial. The jury is still out as to whether all people who are female-bodied have one or whether they are even a thing. This is due to the fact that not all female-bodied people are able to find their G-spot or experience ejaculation. My advice? Don't worry about whether you or your partner have a G-spot. Focus on whether you're having positive and pleasurable consensual sex.

Menstruation

A female-bodied person does not start **menstruating** until she starts puberty. For a female-bodied person, the average starting age for menstruation is between ages nine to fifteen-years-old. Menstruation will start when the ovaries start producing the hormones estrogen and progesterone.

Whether you have one or not, it's important to know what a period is and what female bodies go through when they have periods.

Did you know that the female **menstrual cycle** refers to the period of time from the first day of one **period** to the first day of the next? A normal menstrual cycle can be as short as 21 days or longer than 35 days. On average, though, it lasts 25–30 days. It isn't just when a female-bodied person has their period, which is when a small amount of blood, other fluids, and tissue leave the uterus about once a month beginning at puberty. The fluid leaves a female-bodied person slowly, usually over the course of three to eight days. At the beginning of the period, the blood may look a little brown or rust-colored. This can also be true at the end of the period. The **flow** (how much and how quickly) can also change throughout the period. This is why there are different sizes of tampons and pads (more on what those are in a minute). It's also pretty normal for a female-bodied person to **spot** at the beginning or end of the period. Basically, this may mean that you see a little bit of blood on your clothes but then the actual period or heavier bleeding doesn't start for a few days. It's also normal for a female-bodied person to have spotting in between her periods.

It's pretty normal for a female-bodied person's period to change from month to month, especially when she is younger and menstruation is new to her body. A female-bodied person will stop having her period during pregnancy. And when a female-bodied person becomes older (usually between forty-five to fifty-five years old, but this is different for every person), the period will stop altogether, and this is called **menopause**.

There are some female-bodied people who have some bleeding or spotting while they are pregnant and this can be confused as a period. But vaginal bleeding while pregnant is not the same as menstruation.

So, it basically sounds like a female-bodied person should just expect to bleed, like, all the time. Not at all! The longer you have your period, the more familiar you will become with what your body's rhythm is. When you start menstruating, you might want to track it. There are apps that can help, or you can use a good old-fashioned calendar or notebook. Tracking can help you determine what your body's rhythm is, and therefore determine if something isn't normal for you. You can also determine whether your period is late and it can help you have a general idea of when your period will happen again.

A lot of female-bodied people get concerned with whether their period is normal. Remember, each person is different. Also, there are some perfectly normal things that can influence your body's period and make it seem "not normal" and even lead to you skip a month of your period. Stress, excessive exercise, and rapid weight gain or loss can affect the menstrual cycle. If you're finding that your period is "off" from your normal rhythm and you have been sexually active, you will definitely want to take a pregnancy test and consider getting testing for STIs. If you are not pregnant and your period continues to be abnormal for you, talk to a health care provider.

Some female-bodied people have clues about when they are about to start bleeding. These symptoms are commonly referred to as **PMS**, which stands for Premenstrual Syndrome. These range from bloating in the belly (the stomach feels full and may be hard, and clothes might not fit like they used to), to swelling in the fingers, hands, or feet, or cramps either in the stomach area (or a little lower) or back. Often using ibuprofen and a heating pad or taking a warm bath can help with the cramping you might feel (either before or during your period). Some female-bodied people get more **acne** (zits or pimples) and some feel more emotional (angry or sad) or experience quick fluctuations between feelings. As you get older, these symptoms will become pretty predictable. But remember, no one can tell just by looking at you or talking to you that you're having your period. And, your period shouldn't keep you from doing what you enjoy. If your period is so heavy that you find you have to change your pad or tampon more than once every two hours regularly, you should consult your health care provider.

If you find you're in a lot of pain, bleeding so heavily you feel like you can't do your normal activities, or feel so depressed or sad that you're having thoughts about suicide or hurting yourself, please talk to your health care provider. There are lots of things that can be done to help relieve your symptoms and get you back to feeling "normal." There are many female-bodied people who use **hormonal birth control** to help with the symptoms of PMS. For more on what hormonal birth control is, go to chapter 14.

When female-bodied people have their periods, most people use pads, tampons, and/or a menstrual cup to contain the blood exiting the vagina and help to keep their clothes from getting stained. Tampons and pads all come in different sizes and shapes. These are for the variations of your flow (ranging from heavy to light). Your body will likely feel

83

best when you use the right size to match your flow. Using something small or "light" when you have a heavy flow will mean you'll need to change it more often than the directions state. Using something that is meant for a heavy flow when you aren't having a heavy flow is fine as long as you change them according to the directions.

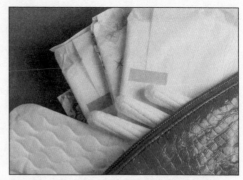

There are so many brands and styles to choose from!

Tampons and pads can be found pretty easily. They are sold in grocery stores, pharmacies, and convenience stores. Menstrual cups are a little harder to come by. There are a couple different brands, but the most well-known are Diva Cups. Here's a great website to order them: divacup.com. Whenever you start using something new, there's going to be a learning curve. Be patient with yourself! All of these products come with directions and usually have diagrams to help you understand the right placement.

ALL THE PERIOD GEAR

Tampons

Tampons are most commonly made out of cotton and fit inside the vagina. They act like a sponge by soaking up the menstrual blood when it leaves the uterus through the cervix. Most people can't feel them when they are inside. If they are uncomfortable, they might not be inserted correctly. Most tampons come with an applicator and this helps to insert the tampon and place it where it will be most effective. Tampons cannot fall out of the vagina. Remember? It's a muscle, so it works to keep the tampon inside.

If you decide you want to give tampons a try, remember to read the directions first. You will want to make sure your hands are clean and then get comfortable. When you're first using tampons, you might feel more comfortable lying down. Or maybe you will feel more comfortable squatting or putting one leg up, like with your foot on the edge of the toilet. You'll just need to try it out and see what works. Once you're in position, you open the package and if the tampon is in the applicator, insert the entire applicator into the vagina. Once inserted, you push the applicator up and that positions the tampon next to your cervix. There are tampons that don't come with applicators. Neither one is better than the other, it's just what you're most comfortable with. If you choose to use a tampon that doesn't come with an applicator, then you use your finger to push the tampon into place. If you find you're having challenges, don't be embarrassed to ask your mom or sister or aunt (someone you trust) to show you how to do it.

- Using tampons is not the same as having sex and does not mean you are not a "virgin" anymore! (Refer to page 121 for more on this.)

- You can pee with a tampon in! (Remember, they are different parts of the female body.)

- Neither tampons or applicators should be flushed down the toilet—it's bad for the sewer system.

- Using a tampon shouldn't hurt. Using one with an applicator (especially plastic) can help you feel more comfortable.

- You can wear tampons in the water!

- Some tampons come scented. First of all, if you are concerned with smell when using a tampon, changing it more often than the directions suggest may help. Secondly, the scents don't really help. And finally, many female-bodied people have an allergic reaction or sensitivity to the perfume used. My advice? Steer clear.

You want to change your tampon every 3–6 hours (but double check the directions with the kind you use). When you are ready to change, or discard your tampon, there is a string you can gently pull on to help bring the tampon out of the body. You can use tampons and pads together for added protection, and you can even wear tampons at night (but no more than 8 hours) if you want. And ta-da! That's the scoop about tampons!

Pads

Pads are also typically made out of cotton. They have a sticky backing so they can stay put in your underwear. Some pads are thick, some are long, some are

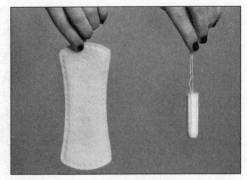

If you're using a tampon, it's a good idea to use a light pad or panty liner in case there is some leakage.

thin, some have "wings," and some are specially designed for thong underwear. Pads come in all these varieties because every body is different and what works for your bestie may not work for you. Some people really like pads because they aren't comfortable putting something inside their vagina. Some people don't like pads because they might feel bulky or like "wearing a diaper." You've got to do what feels comfortable for you! And remember, you can use a tampon and pad together for extra protection.

If you want to try using a pad, the easiest way to do this is to sit on the toilet so that your underpants are accessible. You'll want to peel off the plastic backing that is covering the sticky part and then take the sticky part of the pad and press it in to the crotch of the underpants (the part of the underpants that would normally be touching your vulva). Just like with a tampon, you need to change your pad often (depending on what thickness of pad you're using and what your flow is like). When you're done with your pad, wrap it up in toilet paper and throw them away.

SIDENOTE:

- Do not flush pads down the toilet, or you might cause a backup—eek!

- You can't wear a pad in the water. Scented pads? Not worth it. The best way to help with smell is to change your pad often and wash the vulva regularly.

Menstrual Cups

Menstrual cups are fairly new to the scene of period management. They are a great option for those who are trying to be more ecofriendly and ultimately save

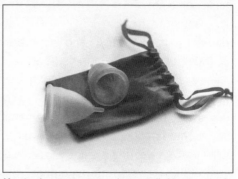

Menstrual cups are a very environmentally friendly option for female-bodied people during their period.

money because they can be reused. Menstrual cups are like little bowls that fit snugly in your vagina (remember, it's a muscle!) and collect the blood as it flows through the cervix—so, it's placed in the vagina as close to the cervix as you can get it. Menstrual cups don't have applicators, so you would need to use your fingers to make sure it's in place. Even though they are flexible and bigger than tampons, most people say they can't feel the cup when it is in the vagina.

- Menstrual cups can't fall out of the body (remember: vagina = muscle).
- Menstrual cups can be worn in the water!

Just like with a pad or tampon, before you use them, read the directions. The use of a menstrual cup is really similar to using a tampon—you need to get your body into a comfortable position. This can be squatting or sitting on the toilet—you gotta do you. You then fold or squeeze the cup to make it smaller, to more easily fit inside the vaginal opening. It may not feel comfortable going in, but it shouldn't hurt. If you're having any problems, remember to talk to someone you trust like your mom, aunt, or sister. Menstrual cups can definitely take more practice than using a tampon or pad, and you need to feel comfortable with your body. You can keep a menstrual cup in up to 12 hours. But just because it can stay inside your vagina for 12 hours doesn't mean it should. If it starts leaking, you will want to take it out and empty the contents in the toilet.

If you want to take the menstrual cup out, you put your fingers into your vagina and grab the cup. By gently squeezing the cup, you can make it smaller than the walls of the vagina and pull it out without spilling it. Remember, menstrual cups can be washed and reused. If you need to get rid of it, though, you want to wrap it up and put it in the trash (not down the toilet!).

AUTHOR'S NOTE:

Language is a powerful tool that sex educators are hyper-aware of, as it's one way we can ensure conversations and teachings are as inclusive and stigma-free as possible. We are always learning, as our intention is to ensure all people get the information they need to make decisions about their health and behavior. Because of this, language is constantly being evaluated and updated to be as inclusive as possible. Some people believe that terms such as "male-bodied" and "female-bodied" are not the most inclusive, because they inadvertently ascribe a gender lens and imply that all male- or female-identified people have the same body parts. Some people suggest using language such as "person with a penis" and "person with a vagina" instead. For the purposes of this publication, the author has chosen to use the language of "male-bodied" and "female-bodied" because they are more commonly understood terms. It is not the author's intent to exclude any individual with the use of this terminology.

8

KEEPING YOUR PARTS HEALTHY

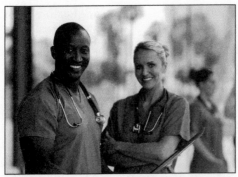

Medical professionals are here to help you. They can answer your questions and check to make sure you're healthy. They can't help you if you don't speak up and tell them the truth though. Make sure you give your medical professional the whole truth so that they can offer you the best medical advice.

Knowing the medically accurate terminology and what is "normal" can help you to take care of your body. If you know what is normal for your body, you can proactively get medical care if you need it. Knowing about your own body can also help you make decisions about your sexual health, like when and what kind of STI (Sexually Transmitted Infections) testing you might need and what kind of contraception you might need.

KEEPING THE MALE BODY HEALTHY

If you're male-bodied, you will need to check your testicles regularly (like once a month). You want to feel the testicles through the scrotum to make sure they are round, you don't feel any lumps and one is not excessively bigger than the other. (Remember: it's normal to have two differently sized testicles, but if that increases or changes, you will want to consult a health care provider as teens can—rarely—get testicular cancer.) Your health care provider will also check your testicles at your annual exams. But since they only see you once per year, you're going to be a better source of information to tell the provider whether they have changed at all.

Additionally, a male-bodied person should seek medical advice if there is ever a sharp pain in the testicles or penis, excessive itchiness, or if bumps develop. But don't freak out if you notice something different happening! There are lots of common things that can cause a change in the male body. The most common is a fungal infection called "jock itch." So how do you prevent getting something like jock itch? Make sure you shower regularly, especially after you have sweated a lot. You will also want to make sure you wash your sports gear in between uses.

Basically, get checked out by a health care provider and do it when you first notice the – whatever it is. The sooner you go in and talk to a health

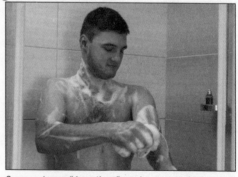

Common issues "down there" can be prevented with proper care, including keeping the bits and parts clean.

care provider, the sooner you can get treatment and start feeling better mentally and physically. Remember, your health care provider is there to help you.

KEEPING THE FEMALE BODY HEALTHY

You know all those commercials out there for douches? Maybe not, but basically it is a liquid that has been created to help women "clean out" their vaginas. Bottom line? Your

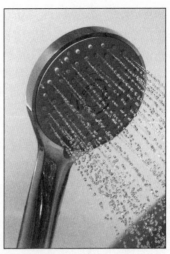

Worried about smell? Regularly bathing with soap is all you need!

body is pretty magnificent and usually does a really good job of taking care of itself. Same goes for the vagina. The vagina is a "self-cleaning" organ. Your normal discharge that you have when you aren't bleeding? (Yeah, the stuff in your underwear.) That is how your vagina cleans itself and keeps itself healthy. Just leave it alone and let it do its job. There is no reason to douche and, in fact, douching can lead to vaginal infections like yeast infections. If you're truly concerned about your vagina's odor, shower often. In fact, even if you aren't concerned about odor, shower. Showering and washing your vulva is really important in keeping yourself healthy.

Another thing you will want to remember for good self-care is to change your tampon and/or pad often. Again, this strategy can help you control your odor and cleanliness. If you're really worried or feeling self-conscious, go get yourself checked out by a health care professional. Even if nothing is "wrong," you will have had a great conversation with your health care provider, and you will have learned more about your body. Win-win!

Speaking of a health care provider, a female-bodied person should start seeing a health care provider who specializes in female anatomy and reproductive health care sometime around the age of twenty-one. The person absolutely can see this provider sooner, but if you haven't, make an appointment. I promise there is nothing to be nervous about!

What's the deal with shaving? Does it help with keeping yourself clean? Short answer? Nope. There is a lot of talk out there about shaving pubic hair. Bottom line: shaving or not shaving is a personal preference and has absolutely nothing to do with cleanliness. Do what you like and are comfortable with. There is no right or wrong when it comes to shaving pubic hair.

What to expect in an exam

Let's face it. Going to the doctor is never much fun, but it's really important! People with female bodies should plan on going to a gynecologist or female health care provider like Planned Parenthood one time per year starting around the age of twenty-one for their annual exam, which includes a pelvic exam. Of course, if you think you have a problem, you will want to go sooner. Or, if you're thinking of becoming sexually active, a chat with the gynecologist or Planned Parenthood staff can help you determine what is going to be the best protection for you.

Female-bodied people will need to get an annual exam, well, annually (that's every year). The health care provider will determine what parts of the pelvic exam you need based on your risk factors (assessed through questions) and history.

Depending on whom you decide to visit, each health care provider's exam room is going to look a little different (and likely, the exam room is going to be a lot more comfortable than the picture here). But I wanted to show you something to give a general idea of what to expect. When you go into the exam room, someone will take your pulse and blood pressure. They will probably have you stand on a scale to get your weight. They'll also have you stand against a measuring tape to see how tall you are. And then they are going to ask you a lot of questions, questions about what kind of sex you have or are thinking about having. Again, this can be a little uncomfortable, but it's really important that you tell the truth. If you're sexually active, you've got to disclose what sexual behaviors you engage in and with whom (male- or

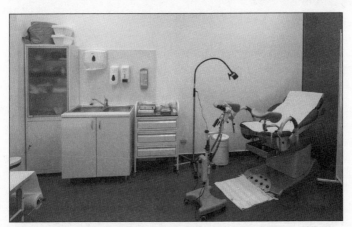

When a female-bodied person gets a gynecological exam, they will be examined on a table similar to this one. Each gynecological exam table has stirrups for the female-bodied person's feet so that they can be comfortable as they spread their legs wide enough for the medical professional to examine the external female genitalia as well as comfortably examine the inside of the vagina and the pelvis, including the uterus.

female-bodied people), whether you use alcohol or drugs, whether you smoke, and when your last period was. You're going to want to be honest, even if you feel uncomfortable answering the questions. The health care provider is not there to judge you or arrest you if you're involved in something illegal. They are trying to assess how to offer you the best medical care.

Unfortunately, I can't guarantee your experience with your health care provider will be free from judgment. It should be. But health care providers are people too. And, as you know, everyone has their own values about behaviors. If the health care provider is any good, they will be able to provide you with care free from their personal values. If they don't? Don't continue to see them. Obviously, if you live in an area where there are lots of options for providers then you have a lot more flexibility. But a lot of people don't have options because there are a limited number of providers or maybe you have insurance or self-pay limitations. In that case, you will need to be a strong advocate for yourself and ensure you balance keeping yourself safe with getting the care you need to stay healthy and make informed decisions.

Back to what to expect at the visit . . .

A pelvic exam is going to require you to get undressed. If the pelvic exam is part of your annual exam, they will probably have you completely undress and have you wear this super cute (insert sarcasm) gown made out of either paper or cloth. If it isn't part of your annual exam, you will probably just get undressed from the waist down. Either way, once you've undressed you will sit on the exam table and drape a sheet (again either paper or cloth) over the lower half of your body. Once the health care provider comes in, they will ask you to lie down and place your feet in the stirrups (those cup-like thingies at the end of the exam table). You will want to slide yourself down to the edge of the exam table. (The health care provider will tell you to keep scootin' down if you aren't down far enough.) You will want to let your knees move apart and try to relax as much as possible.

Did you know you can see your health care provider and have a pelvic exam even when you're on your period? Of course, you will want to remove any tampon or menstrual cup prior to the examination. If you're having a heavy flow, it may be hard for the health care provider to see the cervix clearly and therefore may ask you to come back once your period has stopped. Also, some female-bodied people feel bloated or crampy during their period. For these reasons, many female-bodied people choose to schedule their annual exam for when they are not having their period.

There are a couple different parts of the exam and each health care provider has their own way of doing things. Generally, you can expect that the health care provider will look at the vulva and opening to the vagina. Remember, that's the external part of the female body. They are looking for any bumps, rashes, abnormal coloring, abnormal discharge or anything else that is unusual. Once they've looked over the external parts, they will look inside the body. They will use what is called a speculum. The speculum is a tool that gets inserted into the vaginal opening after it has been lubricated. It sort of looks like a duck bill. Once it is inserted, the health care provider opens it. Remember that the vagina is a muscle so it will stretch as the speculum opens. It might feel a little uncomfortable or weird, but it shouldn't hurt. If it does, you will want to tell your health care provider. Speculums come in differ-

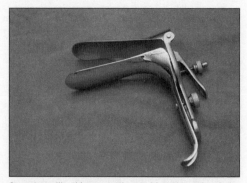

Speculums like this one are inserted into the vagina during an annual gynecological exam. Once inserted, it can hold the walls of the vagina open so that the medical provider can use both of their hands to conduct the exam. Speculums can also be made of clear plastic.

ent sizes, so the health care provider can hopefully make it more comfortable for you. But, of course, the health care provider won't know they need to switch things up unless you tell them.

Once the speculum is in place, the health care provider is going to swab your cervix (the gateway between the vagina and uterus). They will use something that looks like a really long Q-tip and insert it into the open vagina and wipe it against the cervix. Again, this shouldn't hurt, but it might feel a little uncomfortable. The health care provider is collecting cervical cells to send to a lab and make sure they are healthy and normal-looking. This is what is called a pap test. If you have decided to test for certain STIs, the health care provider will do that at this time, too. Again, they will use a Q-tip-looking thing, which they use to gather a sample of your discharge. Again, this sample will be tested in a lab (either on-site or off-site). Once the samples have been collected, the speculum will be removed.

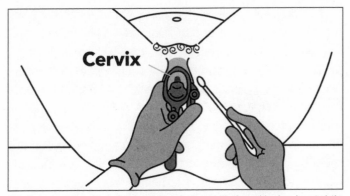

This is a simulation of what it looks like when a medical provider has inserted the speculum into the vagina. In the medical provider's right hand they are holding a swab. This exam can be uncomfortable but is not painful.[11]

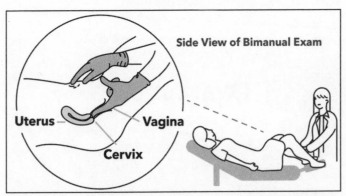

As you can see, the medical provider inserts their fingers inside the vagina to feel the cervix, the inside of the vagina and help them feel the uterus. A medical provider will use lubricant on their fingers to make the experience as comfortable as possible. This, in no way, is the same as the sexual act of "fingering" (when a partner inserts their fingers inside the vagina for sexual stimulation).[12]

11 "What Is a Pelvic Exam? | Questions About Gynecology Exams." Planned Parenthood. Accessed January 17, 2018. http://www.plannedparenthood.org/learn/health-and-wellness/well-woman-visit/what-pelvic-exam.

12 "What Is a Pelvic Exam? | Questions About Gynecology Exams." Planned Parenthood. Accessed January 17, 2018. http://www.plannedparenthood.org/learn/health-and-wellness/well-woman-visit/what-pelvic-exam.

Another part of the exam consists of the health care provider inserting one or two of their gloved fingers into your vagina and, using the other hand, they will press down on the outside of your abdomen. They will lubricate their fingers before insertion. This is how the health care provider checks the size and shape of your uterus, as well as the position of your uterus in your body. If this feels at all tender or painful, you will want to notify your health care provider, as this could be the sign of an infection or something else they will want to look into further. The health care provider is also feeling the size and shape of your ovaries and fallopian tubes to ensure there aren't any cysts or tumors. This part of the exam is called the "bimanual exam."

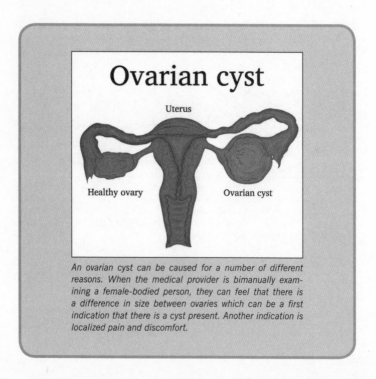

An ovarian cyst can be caused for a number of different reasons. When the medical provider is bimanually examining a female-bodied person, they can feel that there is a difference in size between ovaries which can be a first indication that there is a cyst present. Another indication is localized pain and discomfort.

Finally, your health care provider may do what is called a rectovaginal exam. These types of exams are not as common as the other two exams that have been mentioned. The purpose of this type of exam is to check the health of the anus muscles and the health of the back-side of your uterus. This type of exam often makes people feel like they need to poop—but don't worry! You won't! That feeling is totally normal and doesn't last long. A rectovaginal exam will only be done if your medical provider has deemed that your medical history warrants this additional screen.

Even though the description of the pelvic exam and pap test took a good chunk of ink, the whole exam is actually pretty quick and only lasts a few minutes. Just remember to relax, take deep breaths, and don't be afraid to ask your health care provider to tell you what they are doing (if they don't already) as they are doing it.

TALKING ABOUT THE BODY

• • • • • • • • • •

Questions for teens:

If you are a male-bodied person...
- Are you circumcised or not?
    - a.) Was this something your parents chose?
    - b.) What was their reason for doing so?

- Have you ever had a "wet dream?" Did you talk to anyone about it? Why or why not?

If you are a female-bodied person...

- Have you gotten your period yet?

- Have you talked to your mom or sister or another trusted adult about your period? Or using a tampon, menstrual cup or pad? How'd that go? Do you feel comfortable talking about your period? If you could tell your parent(s) some things about how you feel (either physically or emotionally) about having your period, what would it be?

1.) _____

_____

2.) _____

_____

3.) _____

_____

4.) _____

_____

5.) _____

_____

Questions for parents:

- What is one thing (or more) that you really wish your parents had talked to you about regarding your body?

- Have you ever had a wet dream? What was your experience? What would you like to share with your teen about wet dreams that you wish you had heard from your parents?

- Was there any part of the human anatomy you found surprising?

9

WE ARE ALL DIFFERENT
AND UNIQUE!

Exploration and understanding of gender identity, gender expression, sex assigned at birth, physical attraction, and emotional attraction

We have already talked a little about why I am using the terms "female-bodied" and "male-bodied." As I explained in chapter 5, it's because even though some people, for ex-

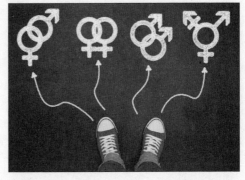

Sexuality for some people is really clear and well defined. Others? Not so much.

ample, have female body parts, they might not identify as "female." The same goes for someone who has male body parts. And then there is whom a person is attracted to and what behaviors they engage in. Often, discussing these issues is referred to as discussing the LGBTQ+ community.

LGBTQ+ stands for: lesbian, gay, bisexual, transgender, and queer, plus so much more. This chapter is really going to take a look at what these terms mean and also what the "plus" is. As with all of this book, there are so many aspects we could dive into, so we are going to keep it as basic as possible to hopefully give you a foundation to build upon. If you are interested in learning more about what the differences are between biological sex, gender identity, and sexual orientation, I suggest checking out the Trans Student Education Resources (TSER) website. There is some really great information, including visuals, which can help both teens and parents make sense of it all.

Let's start with figuring out what biological sex is (or what is also referred to as "sex assigned at birth"). When (just about) every person is born, a doctor or midwife or parent looks at the baby and says, "It's a boy!" Or, "It's a girl!" They are making this statement based on whether they see a vulva or penis (for more on the biological anatomy go to chapter 7). Sometimes, the baby is born with anatomy that is not clearly "male" or "female." This child is "intersex." So, this could be a child who is born with a noticeably large clitoris or lacks a vaginal opening. Or maybe they present as one gender physically but at the chromosomal level, they are actually a different gender. Intersex can also refer to an individual who has a combination of male and female reproductive organs. Bottom line? For most of us, our biological sex or sex assigned at birth isn't ours to define and it is decided by the adults in the room. In a nutshell, that is what biological sex is.

Now that we know what biological sex is, let's discuss gender identity. Gender identity is completely in a person's mind. It's that person's perception of who they are, whether they are female, male, both, or neither. If you think of the biological sex of a person as what is between a person's legs, gender identity is found in the head or brain. Often a person's biological sex lines up with their gender identity. When it does, this person is referred to as "cisgender." But it often doesn't. If this is the case, the person is referred to as transgender. Simply, a transgender person is someone whose biological sex doesn't align with their gender identity. Additionally, a person may not identify as one hundred percent female or one hundred percent male. As with many things in sexuality there is a gender spectrum. And this spectrum is fluid, meaning it can change over time. Because of this, they may identify as "gender queer," "gender fluid," or "gender non-conforming."

The development of gender identity can take several years to develop, and parents and caregivers can usually see a child identifying in one way or the other around the age of six. It isn't uncommon for children six and under to engage in what is called "gender play." Gender play is simply a child trying out different roles traditionally seen as male or female such as wearing high heels or putting on makeup or wearing extremely short hair and a necktie.

How a person chooses to express their gender is called "gender expression." Many people express their gender in a way that matches their gender identity and/or their biological sex. Some people don't. It's important to remember that there is a lot of cultural influence on how a person expresses their gender. For example, if we look at what people put on their bodies—clothing, jewelry, makeup—those things may all signal to the observer that a person is a certain gender.

When it comes to gender, remember that we can't make assumptions about how a person identifies based on how they express themselves. Many things can influence how a person expresses who they are, not just gender.

Finally, let's talk a little about attraction. (Attraction can often be referred to as "orientation.") Attraction is how you feel toward other people. There are two ways people are attracted to others: emotionally and physically. It's important to call out these two components of attraction. Because, to make things even more confusing, a person can be emotionally attracted to both "males" and "females," but only physically attracted to males. Or vice versa. Or any combination thereof, actually. There are labels for all of these types of attractions (this is where we are getting into the LGB part of LGBTQ+). A person can also find that they aren't really attracted to others. When a person isn't attracted to others, the person is called "asexual."

Here's the breakdown (remember, this is about how the person intellectually and emotionally *identifies*):

- Heterosexual, or straight, means that a person is attracted to a different gender. So, a person who identifies as female is attracted to those who identify as male, and vice versa.

- Lesbian, gay, or homosexual means that a person is attracted to the same gender identity as how they identify. A lesbian is a person who identifies as a woman and is attracted to others who identify as women. A person who is gay identifies as male and is attracted to others who identify as male.

- Bisexual means that a person is attracted to both people who identify as male and those who identify as female (regardless of how they identify).

- Pansexual is similar to bisexuality. It means that a person experiences attraction regardless of the other person's gender expression and identity.

- Queer is a generic term that can encompass many different identities and orientations.

- Gender-queer is someone whose gender identity doesn't fit on the spectrum of male or female.

- Asexual means that a person doesn't feel attracted to others or doesn't have sex.

These labels can be helpful to make sense of gender, gender expression and gender identity. But, keep in mind that people are so much more complicated than a simple label. The label might help us to make sense of sexuality, but often, people don't fit cleanly in a certain label. Just remember that attraction is based on how you and your partner *identify*. So, for example, if a male-bodied person does not identify as male, but rather identifies as female, and they are attracted to a male-bodied and male identifying person, their relationship is heterosexual (straight). I told you it can be confusing! It's confusing because sexuality is fluid and influenced by a ton of different factors. Some of these are biological and some are socio-cultural (as in what your family is like, what part of the world you live in, what your community's ideology is . . .). [13] The best thing to do is not make assumptions and recognize that we are all different and beautiful just the way we are!

13 Frankowski, B. L. Sexual Orientation and Adolescents. Pediatrics113, no. 6 (2004): 1827-832. doi:10.1542/peds.113.6.1827.

Hammack, P. The Life Course Development of Human Sexual Orientation: An Integrative Paradigm. Human Development. University of Chicago, 2005.

WE ARE ALL DIFFERENT AND UNIQUE!

CONVERSATION STARTERS . . .

• • • • • • • • • •

The conversation starters are designed to be prompts for having conversations. Feel free to use them in the way that feels right to you.

Questions for Teens to Ask Their Parents

- Have you ever thought about your sexual identity or questioned whom you're attracted to? Have you expressed this to your family, parents, or friends? Why or why not?

- When did you first notice whom you're attracted to?

Questions for Parents to Ask Their Teen

- According to Advocates for Youth and the Marian Wright Edelman Institute, "GLBTQ youth with more rejecting families are eight times more likely to report having attempted suicide, nearly six more times as likely to report high levels of depression, more than three times as likely to use illegal drugs, and three times as likely to be at high risk for HIV and sexually transmitted diseases than GLBTQ youth with less rejecting families."[14] What do you think are some contributing factors to this?

---

14 Advocatesforyouth.org. Accessed January 17, 2018. http://www.advocatesforyouth. org/publications/424-glbtq-youth.

Ryan, C. Supportive families, healthy children: Helping families with lesbian, gay, bisexual, & transgender children. San Francisco, CA: Marian Wright Edelman Institute, San Francisco State University, 2009.

- Did you know that youth of color who are also LG-BTQ+ experience more discrimination and rejection by society as a whole as well as by their communities of color than LGBTQ+ individuals who identify as white? Youth of color are significantly less likely to tell their parents that they are LGBTQ+ than white LGBTQ+ teens. LGBTQ+ teens of color are also more likely to experience higher rates of STI infections and substance use with sex than their white counterparts. Why do you think that might be?

10

SOOOO . . . LIKE, WHAT, EXACTLY, IS SEX?

Now that you know all the parts and the basics of what they do to make a person ready to have sex, let's take a look at what sex is. Everyone has their own definition of sex. Generally speaking, there are three types of sex: vaginal, oral, and anal.

While there are three common forms of sex, there are lots of variations of these activities that can lead to stimulation and pleasure and that some people put in the category of "sex." Some of these activities are relatively low risk for getting an STI or becoming pregnant. Please refer to chapter 10 to dive deeper into what is risky and what is safe when it comes to sexual activity. Some examples of other "sex acts" are dry humping or rubbing genitals over clothes, using fingers to bring a partner to orgasm, and masturbation (including mutual masturbation).

Whether it's a penis, toy, or finger, partners should consider using a condom to protect against STIs.

When you're considering being sexually active it's critical that you think about what you're comfortable doing and how you like to be touched. Being sexually active should be a pleasurable experience for the people involved. Similarly, being sexually active takes a lot of responsibility. As we have discussed, sexual activity has some risk associated with it. Only you can decide what amount of risk you're comfortable taking, and deciding how to mitigate those risks or protect yourself is a critical part of being sexually active.

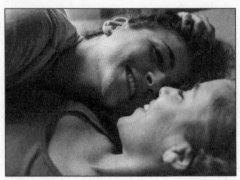

Partners that have the same genitalia can still engage in the three different kinds of sexual activity. (Unless you're both male-bodied, then obviously, you won't be engaging in vaginal sex.)

VAGINAL SEX

Vaginal sex refers to the act of penetrating (inserting) and/ or stimulating the vagina with a penis, finger or toy. Some people call this "hooking up," "doing the nasty," or "getting it on." If a female-bodied person is having vaginal sex with a male-bodied person, they are at risk of pregnancy as well as STIs. We are going to go into how to protect oneself from pregnancy in chapter 14.

ORAL SEX

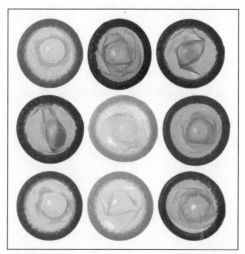

Condoms come in all sorts of different colors, designs and flavors. If you're choosing a condom for oral sex, try a flavored one! Using an unflavored condom may not be as pleasurable for the person giving oral sex. Also, make sure that the condom used isn't lubricated with spermicide as spermicide isn't supposed to be ingested.

Oral sex refers to the act of stimulating the genitals with the mouth and/ or inserting the penis into the mouth. This can be called "going down on someone," "eating some-one out," "giv-ing a blow job," or "giving head." Not everyone engages in oral sex. Some people like it and some don't. Some people like to give another person oral sex, but don't like to have oral sex performed on them and vice versa. It's a personal prefer-ence and decision.

You can get an STI from oral sex, so if you decide to engage in this activity you need to protect yourself and your partner. The best protection for oral sex on a penis is a condom. There are even flavored condoms made just for oral sex! Protecting yourself or your partner when engaging in oral sex on the vulva or anus requires that you use what is a called a dental dam. The dental dam is placed over the vulva or anal opening prior to sexual activity. Unfortunately, both flavored condoms and dental dams are not as readily available as regular condoms, but they can be found online and in sex toy stores.

LUBRICATION

Lubrication during any kind of sex is important. Lubrication helps to reduce friction between body parts. Lubricant is commonly called "lube." When having sex, you should purchase and use lubricant specifically made for sexual activity. You will want to make sure it is a water-based lubricant. Don't use baby oil, olive oil, Vaseline or lotion. These

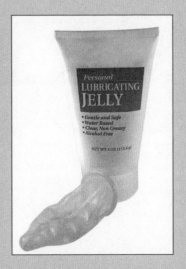

products are not created to be used for sex and can cause irritation. They can even break down the latex of a condom. A lot of condoms come pre-lubricated.

It is especially important to use lube during anal sex to make it feel better and keep a condom from breaking since the anus doesn't produce its own lubricant.

You can buy lubricant at the drugstore, grocery store or sex store.

ANAL SEX[15]

Anal sex refers to the act of penetrating and/or stimulating the anus on either a female- or male-bodied person with a penis, finger, or toy. People engage in anal sex because there are actually a lot of nerve endings in the anus, and for some people, when those nerve endings are stimulated, it feels really good. In fact, the most nerve endings are at the opening of the anus (also called the "butthole"), so it can even feel good when the opening is stimulated (even if there isn't any penetration). Additionally, if a male-bodied person receives anal sex their prostate is stimulated. Remember when we were learning about anatomy? (Go to page 61 if you need a refresher.) The prostate is a gland that produces a fluid that becomes a component of semen. When the prostate is stimulated through penetration it can feel good and lead to orgasm. But anal sex isn't just enjoyable for a male-bodied person. A female-bodied person can also have pleasure with anal sex. They just don't have a prostate to stimulate.

If you decide you want to engage in anal sex, you first need to talk to your partner and get their consent. As with all sex acts, talking about what you want to do is important *before* you actually start having sex. This means you get or give consent on exactly what is going to be put into the anus. And remember, even if your partner gives consent to having anal sex, they can still change their mind. If you start having anal sex and are told to stop, you need to respect their decision. If you want to tell your partner to stop, you can, and they should respect your decision as well.

Once you have obtained consent, you want to go to the

15 Engle, Gigi. 2007. "Everything You Need to Know About Anal Sex." Teen Vogue. July 10, 2017. Accessed January 17, 2018. http://www.teenvogue.com/story/anal-sex-what-you-need-to-know.

store. Even though pregnancy is not going to be a concern, STIs are. Get some condoms to cover whatever is going to be used during anal play. There are a lot of blood vessels as well as feces (or poop particles) present. The best way to stay safe during anal is to use a condom on the penis, finger, or toy and to use a new one each time. (Also, if you're going to switch between anal and either oral or vaginal, use a new condom. You don't want something covered in feces to go into a vagina or mouth as this can make you and/or your partner really sick.)

While you're at the store, buy some lubricant. Lubricant will help to ease the friction caused by inserting something into the anus. This is really important. The anus doesn't produce its own lubrication. In order to make it as pleasurable as possible for both partners, using lubrication can reduce anal tears and the chance that the condom will rip.

If you're new to anal sex, it's important to take it slow. Anal sex can be painful if you go too fast or try to insert something very large without working up to the large object. If the person receiving anal sex isn't relaxed, that can also lead to pain and discomfort. If you and your partner are choosing to use sex toys for anal stimulation, you'll need to make sure they are the toys that are specially designed to insert into the anus. This part is *really* important! The anus is a strong muscle. So, sometimes when things are inserted into it, the anus can sort of pull them into the body. Using a toy specifically designed for anal stimulation will make it impossible for the toy to go too far into the body. These toys have flat bases that prevent them from fully entering the body. If you choose to use a toy not designed for anal sex, you may find yourself needing a visit to the ER, and possibly needing a surgical intervention.

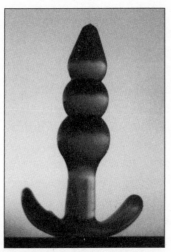

This is just one example of an anal toy. With any anal sex, remember to use lots of lubrication.

Again, some people really enjoy anal sex, but some people don't. And either is fine. Make sure that you know what you want to do and that your partner respects your sexual limits. Sex should always be safe and comfortable for each person involved. If you start to have anal sex (or any kind of sex, really) and it's painful or you don't like it, stop.

Depending on who you talk to, "hooking up" can mean different things. It's a pretty generic term that means the people involved engaged in some kind of casual sexual activity (which can run the gamut from kissing to vaginal, anal, and/or oral sex). The people are not in a romantic relationship together and hookups can happen just the one time or repeatedly with the same partner. According to the Urban Dictionary, "vagueness is its hallmark" so don't make assumptions on the type of sexual behavior that was engaged in if someone tells you they "hooked up."

WHAT'S AN ORGASM?

An orgasm is a pleasurable release of built-up tension that can happen from sexual stimulation. You might have heard an orgasm referred to as "cumming" or "coming." When a person experiences an orgasm, it's an intense and good feeling. Often, people feel warm all over, their heart starts beating very fast, and their genitals will spasm. While orgasms feel good, they aren't the end goal of having sex. Many people get pleasure from doing different sexual acts that don't end in orgasm. Don't worry if you're sexually active and do not orgasm, because that can happen. If you're really worried about the orgasm part of sex, it might make sex less enjoyable.

The Male-Bodied Orgasm

Male-bodied individuals can often orgasm faster than female-bodied individuals. Typically, a male will ejaculate when they orgasm.

The Female-Bodied Orgasm

For a female-bodied person, the stimulation of the clitoris can more frequently lead to orgasm. It's possible for a woman to ejaculate during orgasm as well. A slang term for a female-bodied person ejaculating is "squirting," and the fluid can look very similar to urine, or pee. There have been some studies around this, and the verdict is still out as to what the actual composition of the fluid is. Regardless of what the fluid is, know that most women don't ejaculate, but all bodies are different, so whether you do or not, it's totally normal.

WHAT DOES IT MEAN TO BE A VIRGIN?[16]

The term "virgin" has been used around the world to define a person, especially a female-bodied person, who has not had penis-to-vagina sex. Anatomically speaking, a "virgin" would be someone whose hymen is still intact the first time they have penis-to-vagina sex. What is a hymen, you ask? Well, it's a thin membrane of skin that stretches across the vagina (inside the body). (Refresher on page 61.)

The term *virgin* is riddled with controversy. First of all, not everyone has penis-to-vagina sex. And, historically, "losing your virginity" has only applied to heterosexual, penis-to-vagina sex. So, there's that. But also, virginity or "being a virgin" has absolutely nothing to do with a medical condition (contrary to many people's belief). It's actually a social construct. Many people believe that as long as the hymen is intact, the female-bodied person can be considered a virgin. You've probably heard stories about the wedding night and the bride and groom bringing out the bedding to "prove" the wedding was "consummated" (meaning the male-bodied person and female-bodied person had penis-to-vagina sex)? So, yeah, historically that happened (people actually wanted to see the female-bodied person's blood—I don't know, people had lots of antiquated notions back then). But stick with me here. That "proof"? It's totally *not* proof!

The hymen can actually be broken in lots of ways that have nothing to do with sex. If you use a tampon, it could break the hymen. If you fall while riding a bike, the hymen could break. If you ride horses, the hymen could break. Some female-bodied people have really thick hymens that

16 Wischhover, Cheryl. 2017. "How To Know If Your Hymen Is Broken: Facts About Your Virginity." *Teen Vogue*. November 08, 2017. Accessed January 17, 2018. http://www.teenvogue.com/story/facts-about-hymen-and-virginity.

are harder to break, while others have thin membranes of skin that break super easily. Shocker—every person's body is different. And yes, sometimes, the hymen breaks the first time you have penis-to-vagina sex or the first time the vagina is penetrated sexually.

P.S.: There is also research out there that shows that the hymen may not "break" at all. That is, it actually stretches with sex. There is also research that shows that as a female-bodied person ages, their hymen shrinks and is almost impossible to detect after 25. And if that wasn't confusing enough, there are plenty of female-bodied people out there who aren't even born with hymens. There sure is a lot that isn't understood about such an "important" tissue. Sheesh!

So now that we know there isn't a true medical state of being that entails virginity, what about the cultural or societal definition? Well, we've already covered the fact that not everyone has penis-to-vagina sex. So, are those people always considered virgins? Does "losing your virginity" also encompass the first time you have oral or anal sex? What about masturbation? Are you a virgin if you have never orgasmed? What if you were forced to have sex before you were ready or before you wanted to?

I'm not saying you can't use the term *virgin*, but I am asking you to think about what using that term implies and how it affects how you perceive yourself. Society and different cultures have stigmatized virginity in various ways. In some societies, someone who is considered a virgin is seen as "pure" and untouched. If a female loses their virginity outside of marriage, they are considered dirty, impure, and shameful. Sometimes, if a female has had sex outside of marriage, she is even labeled a "slut." Conversely, in some social groups, being considered a virgin can be viewed as negative and stigmatizing. Most commonly, it is the male who is stigmatized if they remain a virgin, and there can be a great amount of peer pressure for a male to "lose their virginity." But with whom? If they are heterosexual and have sex with a female, that female is shamed while the male is praised. If they are homosexual and have sex with the same sex, did they "lose their virginity"? It's such an antiquated term that has a lot of shame associated with it. It's a term that implies a person cannot be a sexual being unless they are married and in a heterosexual relationship. And for some people, it's a bad thing while for other people it's a good thing. Honestly, it's all kinda BS. Whether you identify as a virgin or not, or want to use that label or not, it's no one's business but your own. If you choose to have sex "outside of marriage," you aren't a bad person. You made a choice about your sexual behavior (if indeed it was a choice). That's it.

11

MASTURBATION: THE BASICS

Masturbation basically means self-pleasuring that involves touching your genitals and often (but not always) leads to orgasm. Masturbation is doing things to your body that you like and figuring out what things feel good to you. Masturbation is a private act that should be done, well, in private. It's commonly done by yourself, but you can also masturbate with a partner. Masturbation is a safe sexual activity that feels good, helps you learn about what you like and don't like sexually, and can be done whether or not you have a partner. When masturbating, a person stimulates the genitals and other erogenous zones (places on the body that feel good to be touched, like the nipples, for example) either with their hands or a sex toy to achieve climax or orgasm. Some people use pornography (see page 35) or other visual or auditory stimuli for arousal. Again, different people are aroused by different things.

Sex toys aren't just for masturbation and can be used with a partner as long as you have consent. In fact, many toys are designed to use with a partner. If you're interested in learning more about sex toys, I encourage you to visit beVibrant.com. This company only sells body safe products.

Masturbation is not "bad" or "good"—it's another way to enjoy sexual activity. It isn't right for everyone, so again, you need to decide if it is right for you. For a male-bodied person, masturbation can involve any part of the body but primarily the penis, scrotum and/or anus. For a female-bodied person, masturbation can include any part of the body but primarily the breasts, vagina, clitoris, and/or anus. When a person masturbates, the human response system will operate as it would if the person were engaging in the sexual behavior with a partner.

When masturbating, make sure you're choosing objects to masturbate with that are safe. Don't put things inside your body that can hurt you (like glass or sharp objects). The anus and vagina are sensitive so if you're choosing to masturbate using something other than your hands, make sure it doesn't contain chemicals or dangerous materials.

If you're using sex toys to masturbate, make sure you keep them clean! Use a gentle soap to wash your sex toy after every use or you could end up getting a nasty infection (like a yeast infection) and those aren't any fun. If you have used a sex toy and think you got an infection (you notice something is going on with your genitals that shouldn't: like a rash, discharge, smell or itchiness) go get checked out by a medical professional. Don't use the toy again without cleaning it because you'll just get the infection back. Some sex toys are made out of really bad materials, so do your research before buying! I can't stress this enough! Don't put something unsafe in your body! If you choose to ignore my warning and do put something in your body that you shouldn't and you develop a problem, get medical help! It might be embarrassing, but it's way better to be safe than sick.

Masturbation as a Male-Bodied Person

When a male-bodied person masturbates, the penis will become erect and the scrotum will contract. Using a toy or hands and often a form of lubrication, the male-bodied person will usually pleasure themselves until they ejaculate. Because of the fluid that will leave the body, it's important to contain the fluid upon ejaculation. Remember, this fluid will contain sperm and if you have an STI, it will contain that too. Some people use condoms to contain the ejaculate while others use a towel or tissue. Just as long as you dispose of it properly. Ejaculate can be sticky, so be respectful and make sure you clean up after yourself.

> **FUN FACT:** You will never run out of semen. Your body will keep making more! So, it doesn't really matter how many times you ejaculate.

A male-bodied person can also masturbate by stimulating their prostate through their anus. Typically, this happens with the hand or a sex toy. As I have already stated, use a sex toy that is designed for anal sexual activity! Do not use a sex toy that has a possibility to go somewhere else in the body—you don't want to have to worry about fecal matter going into a vagina or mouth at another time. If a male-bodied person is using a sex toy, they will want to make sure it's cleaned after every use so that the risk of infection goes down.

Masturbation as a Female-Bodied Person

When a female-bodied person masturbates, their nipples will become erect, the clitoris will fill with blood and become sensitive and the vagina will produce lubrication. Whether using the hand, fingers, or a toy, these items have the possibility of going inside the body. Therefore, it's important that the object being used is clean. And, I am going to stress this again: *use something especially designed for sexual activity.* This is true for sex toys as well as lubrication. Using household materials can be dangerous or cause an irritation or infection that could lead to a doctor visit.

A female-bodied person can also ejaculate when they orgasm through masturbation. This isn't as common as it is with a male-bodied person, but it's possible. Also, a female-bodied person can masturbate by stimulating their anus, as well. Again, the same guidelines are suggested as on page 117: use body-safe materials and make sure things that go in the anus are just used in the anus and not put into the vagina, as this can lead to infection.

A female-bodied person does not have to use penetration to masturbate. A female-bodied person can achieve orgasm through clitoral stimulation only. This is why there are sex toys like the "bullet," which is a vibrator specifically designed just to stimulate the clitoris.

There is no right or wrong way to masturbate. Again, masturbation is about what feels good to you. You can do it as often as you like—it's a safe behavior that causes pleasure and helps you to understand what you do and don't like to do sexually. Not everyone masturbates. Some people masturbate every day. Some people just masturbate once a week or once a month. Again, this is personal preference. If you're worried you masturbate too much, talk to someone about it—like your parent. While masturbation might be one of those things people get embarrassed talking about, I'm gonna bet almost everyone has done it!

CONVERSATION STARTERS...

• • • • • • • • • •

The conversation starters are designed to be prompts for having conversations. Feel free to use them in the way that feels right to you.

Questions for Teens to Ask Their Parents

- Did you ever masturbate when you were younger?

- Did you ever have a wet dream?

Questions for Parents to Ask Their Teens

- Do you need anything to make sure you are being safe when masturbating?

- This is a good time to also lay out any expectations you might have around masturbation. For example, ask your teen to masturbate in private, ensure a younger sibling can't find sex toys by accident, and/ or ensure that bedding or towels are washed.

12

HONEST. IT'S NOT THAT SCARY. LET'S TALK ABOUT RISKS

When (and if) you decide to become sexually active, there are lots of things to think about: what kind of sexual activity you want to engage in, what level of risk you're comfortable taking (see chapter 10), what type of relationship you're in. These are all great things to discuss with your partner.

How do you know if an activity is low risk, medium risk, or high risk? Think about the sexual behaviors that lead to pregnancy and/or STI transmission. All sexual behaviors fall on a continuum that ranges from low risk to high risk. The lowest risk means that there isn't a strong chance of becoming pregnant or getting an STI when you engage in that behavior. Different behaviors have different risks, but they depend on whether or not you're working to mitigate (or lower) those risks. If you and your partner decide to try a certain behavior, like oral sex, your risk of pregnancy is low. However, your risk of STI transmission is high if you don't protect yourself properly by using condoms and/or dental dams. If you use condoms and/or dental dams when engaging in oral sex, you and your partner have decreased your risk for STI transmission. So, something that was a high risk without proper protection has now become medium risk.

NO-RISK BEHAVIORS

Let's start with the most effective forms of contraception and the activity, or lack thereof, that will ensure you have the lowest risk of becoming pregnant or getting an STI. This method is very straightforward—not having sex. It's true. If you really don't want to risk getting pregnant or getting another person pregnant and don't want to risk the transmission of an STI, don't have sex. This is called **abstinence**. A person can choose to be abstinent at any point in their life, regardless of whether they have had sex before. But abstinence only works when you talk to your partner about it and you're both on the same page.

Abstinence, or not engaging in sexual activity, is going to be the sure-proof way to not get an infection or become pregnant, but being one hundred percent abstinent isn't always what people choose to do. Often, people choose to not have sex but engage in other sexual activity like touching or kissing. Don't get me wrong—not having sex is going to be your best bet, especially if you aren't sure you're ready, but if you're in a romantic relationship with someone, you better make sure they know what you mean by "not having sex."

That's right, communicate with your partner about what you are or aren't willing to do. And you need to do it before you start getting busy. Setting up expectations with your partner will take out the guess work and make the experience more enjoyable for you both. It's pretty common for people to go slowly and try different sexual behaviors, become comfortable with those, and then move onto new behaviors that might make them feel more vulnerable. The more you're invested in your partner, the readier you'll both be to engage in higher risk behaviors because there is trust established. If you don't trust your partner, you probably aren't ready for those behaviors that have more risk associated with them. So, if you feel ready to do something new, don't spring that on your partner in the moment. Talk about it beforehand and get their consent for the behavior (refer to chapter 16 for more on consent).

LOW-RISK BEHAVIORS

Okay, so let's say you and your partner have talked and one hundred percent abstinence isn't for you. There are still lots of activities you can engage in with your partner that have low risk associated with them. Kissing, whether on the lips or body, is pretty safe as long as it doesn't involve the mouth on the genitals (that's actually a high-risk behavior). Touching (again, except on the genitals unless it's over the clothes) is also a low-risk behavior. Holding hands, hugging, mutual masturbation (when both you and your partner masturbate at the same time) are all pretty risk-free activities.

When you decide to have sex, no matter what kind of sex you're having, you need to protect yourself. Anytime you're engaging in sexual activity when fluids might be present, you need to use the proper protection. Sexual activity does have certain risks. Some behaviors have fewer risks than others. We are going to talk about what the risks are and how you can mitigate those risks. And, yeah, there's a continuum here, too.

MEDIUM-RISK BEHAVIORS

Medium-risk behaviors basically mean that your risk has increased because you're coming into contact with fluids, but the fluids are not entering another person's body. So, there is still a risk of pregnancy or getting an STI, but it's still pretty minimal or unlikely, and there are things you can do to minimize that risk even further.

An example of medium-risk behaviors is digital or toy stimulation of a partner. Digital or toy stimulation is using either your fingers or a toy to bring your partner pleasure and maybe orgasm. Because this activity will likely lead to ejaculation and vaginal secretions, the people involved can use protection to ensure that the fluids do not get on their partner. For example, using a condom on a male-bodied person will contain the ejaculate or semen. If you don't have a condom, turning away from your partner when you ejaculate can ensure that no fluids get on your partner. It's also important that if you're engaging in digital stimulation (using the fingers or hands), the fingers/hands are clean before engaging in the activity. Then a good wash is important afterwards. If you use a sex toy, it needs to be washed in between each use with soap that is specially designed for the sex toys. If soap is left on the toy, it could irritate the vagina or anus, leading to an infection or rash.

HIGH-RISK BEHAVIORS

Having sex is going to be your high-risk behavior. And that's all kinds of sex (oral, anal, and vaginal). If you're curious about what those types of sex are, please refer to chapter 10.

A lot of people think that oral or anal sex is safer than vaginal sex because there is no risk of pregnancy. Which is true. If a penis isn't going inside the vagina, the risk of pregnancy goes *way* down. But anal sex and oral sex have just as much risk associated with them as vaginal sex does when it comes to STIs. In order to reduce the risk involved in these behaviors, male-bodied people should always use a condom and female-bodied people should always use a dental dam. If two female-bodied people are engaging in sexual activity, they are still at high risk even if they aren't using a penis. As we talked about in the medium-risk section, fluids are still present. So, two female-bodied people need to use proper protection as well. A condom on a sex toy (that is changed for each person and sex act) or a dental dam on the opening of the anus or vagina can also reduce the risk of infection. We are going to talk more about how to keep ourselves safe in chapter 14. Let's first figure out what we need to be safe from.

CONVERSATION STARTERS . . .

• • • • • • • • • •

The conversation starters are designed to be prompts for having conversations. Feel free to use them in the way that feels right to you.

Questions for Teens to Ask Their Parents

- Do you have any concerns for me when it comes to being sexually active?

- What do you think the biggest risk is for me? Why?

Questions for Parents to Ask Their Teens

- What concerns you most about being sexually active? Why?

- What can I do to help you be safe? (Make sure to outline what you are comfortable doing for them to help reduce the risk. If your teen is female-bodied, are you comfortable taking them to a health care facility to get on contraception? Can you help ensure your teen is tested for STIs regularly? What about the HPV vaccine?)

13

BUGS AND VIRUSES: SEXUALLY TRANSMITTED INFECTIONS

Let's discuss what Sexually Transmitted Infections or STIs are. (Heads up – these are sometimes called STDs, or Sexually Transmitted Diseases. We are going to call them STIs because not all of them are actual diseases.) STIs are infections or diseases that are typically passed through sexual behaviors, primarily oral, anal and vaginal sex. Some kinds of STIs can be passed through skin to skin contact. And sometimes STIs can be passed by sharing needles (used for drugs, piercings, or tattoos) or from a woman to her baby during childbirth. Women can also pass some STIs to their babies through breastfeeding. Nearly half of all new cases of STIs in the United States were teenagers and young adults in 2008. That's 9.7 million out of 19.7 million new cases of reported STIs.[17]

You can only get an STI from someone who has one.

17 "Adolescent Sexual and Reproductive Health in the United States." Guttmacher Institute. September 11, 2017. Accessed January 17, 2018. http://www.guttmacher.org/fact-sheet/american-teens-sexual-and-reproductive-health.

Your body can't just create an STI. And you definitely cannot get an STI from holding hands, hugging, sharing a drink (unless you are sharing a drink with someone who has an open sore on their mouth), or sitting on a toilet seat. Also, if a person has an STI, it doesn't mean they are "bad" or "dirty." People primarily get STIs by engaging in sexual activity and not using protection. That's it.

There are three kinds of STIs: parasitic, bacterial and viral. Parasitic STIs are little bugs, or parasites, that live on your body and, with proper treatment, you can get rid of them. Bacterial infections are similar to other bacterial infections you might get (like a sinus infection for example), so they can be cured once proper medication is taken. Viral STIs are not curable, but the symptoms can be treated.

Each STI has different symptoms, but what is most important to remember is that many STIs have *no symptoms at all*. That's right—if a person has an STI, you can't tell just by looking at them. The only way to know if you or your partner have an STI is to get tested, and you can get tested at any health care clinic. If you do have symptoms, you'll notice them around your genitals. Some general symptoms can include soreness, swelling, bumps, sores, rashes, itching, unusual discharge (either increased discharge, a different smell, or a strange color) or bleeding (that is different from a period). If you have some of these symptoms, you will still need to be tested since they could be signs of an STI or another medical problem.

GETTING TO KNOW THE DIFFERENT KINDS OF STIS

As we have already discussed, there are several different STIs. We are going to get to know them a little better in this section. This section is not meant to scare you. Rather, it's important to understand what the risks are associated with STIs so that you can properly protect yourself and advocate for your health with your partner and medical provider. In order to get a general understanding of the STIs you have a risk of transmitting, I organized them according to whether they are parasitic, bacterial or viral. After that, I just organized them alphabetically.

Parasitic STIs

Things to keep in mind about parasitic STIs:

- With proper treatment, you can get rid of them!

- As long as you have the parasite, you can transmit them to your partner, even if you don't see any symptoms.

- Itchiness is the most common symptom.

- The only people who can diagnose them are medical professionals.

- This kind of STI can be passed from one person to another through sexual contact as well as more casual contact like sharing clothes.

Pubic Lice

Commonly called crabs, pubic lice are similar to lice that you might get in the hair on your head, but they are found in the hair around your genitals. (So, while they are both parasites, they are actually different bugs.) Because pubic lice are parasites, they need a host (you) in order to live; they actually eat your blood. Which means that pubic lice can't be picked up from a toilet seat, because they can't live on the toilet seat. (There's no blood on a toilet seat, and if you're choosing to use a toilet seat that is covered in blood, we need to have a different conversation!)

Pubic lice are really easy to catch if your partner has them. In fact, about 3 million people in the U.S. get pubic lice every year.[18] They are most commonly spread through sexual contact. Pubic lice like warm, dark places, like the pubic hair around your genitals. Even if you shave your pubic hair you can still get pubic lice because the little critters get into the roots of the hair and lay their eggs there.

You'll know you have pubic lice because you'll have some pretty intense itching. Sometimes you can even see them. They actually look like tiny little crabs that you might find on the beach. They are typically tan or light gray in color and get darker when they become full of blood. You might notice that your skin looks bruised where the crabs are. Additionally, you could generally feel a little feverish. While pubic lice are most commonly found in pubic hair, they can also live in other coarse hair on the human body like in armpit hair, chest hair, beards, or even eyebrow hair.

The only way you will know for sure if your symptoms are caused by pubic lice is to see a medical professional. The good news is that if you do get pubic lice, you can easily get rid of them and they don't cause any real damage. So, the sooner you get seen by a medical professional, the sooner you can get rid of those little buggers and get rid of the itching and discomfort.

18 Pubic Lice | SexInfo Online. Accessed January 17, 2018. http://www.soc.ucsb.edu/sexinfo/article/pubic-lice.

And, yeah, the concept of having little bugs living on your body might sound gross, but just because someone has pubic lice doesn't mean the person isn't clean or doesn't take care of their body. Only using special medicated soap on the infected area(s) can get rid of pubic lice. Regular soap doesn't cut it. Shaving also doesn't get rid of pubic lice. If someone has pubic lice they must get medication specifically designed to eliminate it as nothing else will work, and if you try to use something that is not specifically designed for pubic lice you could end up doing more damage to your skin.

Scabies

Scabies are similar to pubic lice, only they are little bugs known as mites. Mites are even smaller than pubic lice, but they also live in the genital hair and are transmitted from person to person through sexual contact. Scabies are even more contagious than pubic lice, though, and are pretty common in situations where there are lots of people living together in close quarters (like a prison). Again, you can't get scabies from a toilet seat, and it's really hard to transmit scabies through casual contact like a handshake. But you can sometimes get them from sharing a bath towel or sharing clothes with someone who has scabies.

Similar to pubic lice, scabies make you really itchy, especially at night. People who have scabies also usually have a rash that kind of looks like pimples or little raised red dots. People may also have what look like small, curly lines on their skin near or in the same place as the itching and rash. The symptoms of scabies can come and go, but without medical treatment they are still there. Until you get proper medical treatment, you can still spread them, even if you aren't having symptoms.

Scabies can be found in more areas than pubic lice because they don't necessarily need coarse hair to live. They are found in areas of the body that have less exposure to fresh air like between your fingers, in your knee and elbow creases, under the breasts, on the scrotum or penis, under the butt or in the belly button to name a few.

Bacterial STIs

Things to keep in mind about bacterial STIs:

- With proper treatment, you can get rid of them!

- While you can get rid of the infection, if you live with an STI for a long time, there can be damage done to the body, specifically the reproductive organs (but other organs can be at risk for damage if they are exposed to the infection, for example, your eyes).

- The only people who can diagnose them are medical professionals.

- This kind of STI can be passed from one person to another through the exchange of fluids (pre-ejaculate, ejaculate, vaginal discharge, and blood).

Chlamydia

Chlamydia is one of the most common STIs around. In fact, according to the CDC (the Center for Disease Control), in 2015, 64.3% of all cases of chlamydia were among people aged fifteen to twenty-four years old. That's a 2.5% increase from 2014 to 2015![19] Chlamydia can also be referred to as

---

19 "2015 Sexually Transmitted Diseases Surveillance." Centers for Disease Control and Prevention. Accessed January 17, 2018. http://www.cdc.gov/std/stats15/adolescents.htm.

"the clam." It's spread through unprotected vaginal, anal, and oral sex because it is present in the fluids that are exchanged during sex.

One of the reasons that it's so common is that a lot of people don't experience symptoms and don't get regularly tested. If a person does experience symptoms, they are commonly: pain or burning when peeing, pain during sex, abnormal vaginal discharge, discharge (other than pre-cum, cum or pee) coming out of the penis, pain in the testicles or anus, and blood or pus coming out of the anus. The only way to know for sure whether you have chlamydia is to get tested by a medical provider. If you test positive for chlamydia, the treatment is pretty easy: take antibiotics as prescribed and contact your partners so they can get tested and treated, too.

Gonorrhea

Gonorrhea is just as common as chlamydia. In fact, the rate of reported gonorrhea cases increased 5.2% for persons aged fifteen to nineteen years in 2015.[20] Also called "the clap" or "the drip," a person can only get gonorrhea if they exchange fluids like those exchanged during sexual intercourse or blood. No one gets gonorrhea by kissing or skin-to-skin touch. Some common symptoms of gonorrhea are just like chlamydia: pain or burning when peeing, pain during sex, abnormal vaginal discharge, discharge (other than pre-ejaculate or pre-cum, cum or pee) coming out of the penis, pain in the testicles or anus, and blood or pus coming out of the anus.

Also, just like chlamydia, this is a bacterial infection that many people show no symptoms of having. The only for

---

20 "2015 Sexually Transmitted Diseases Surveillance." Centers for Disease Control and Prevention. Accessed January 17, 2018. http://www.cdc.gov/std/stats15/adolescents.htm.

sure way to know whether you have gonorrhea is to get tested. The good news is that if you test positive for gonorrhea, you can get antibiotics to get rid of it. But, you need to make sure your partner (and all your partners) also gets tested and treated.

Syphilis

A less common STI, syphilis almost completely disappeared, but the Center for Disease Control (CDC) is reporting that they are seeing a comeback of this STI—eek! There are more reported cases of syphilis in adults than teens. But that doesn't mean you're risk-free. In fact, young adults (twenty to twenty-four years old) have the highest rates of this STI.[21]

While syphilis may not be as common as other bacterial STIs, it can be pretty dangerous if it's left untreated. Unfortunately, the symptoms of syphilis are not easy to recognize. Syphilis manifests itself in stages and these stages don't necessarily happen in the same order for everyone. Sometimes they even manifest all at the same time. Additionally, the symptoms of syphilis are similar to some pretty common illnesses so they can sometimes be missed.

The first stage, referred to as the Primary Stage, is when a chancre sore develops on the skin. A chancre is a sore that is typically painless (another reason why it might go unnoticed, especially if it's inside the vagina or anus where it can't be seen). Syphilis chancres are round and can sometimes be "open" and have pus. But a lot of the time they look like a pimple or ingrown hair. And, if it isn't hurting, you might not give it much thought. A person typically will have just one chancre, but it's possible to have several at the same time.

---

21 "STDs in Adolescents and Young Adults." Centers for Disease Control and Prevention. Accessed January 17, 2018. http://www.cdc.gov/std/stats12/adol.htm.

Genital contact with the chancre is one way syphilis is spread. Skin-to-skin contact is hard to protect against since an internal condom, external condom, and even dental dam offer limited skin coverage, but the chancres are really, really contagious. If a person does get a chancre, it's going to show up sometime between three weeks to three months after exposure. Yikes! That's a long time to not know that you have syphilis! And if you're having sex with anyone during that time period, they have been exposed. Bummer.

The chancres will go away after three to six weeks even if you don't do anything about them. This is another reason why this STI is so hard recognize. A lot of the time when people have something different going on with their body, they wait it out. Or they try topical, over-the-counter treatments to help manage the symptoms, waiting to see if they improve. And while that advice is often good with things like a zit or cold, this advice isn't so good with a chancre. Just because the chancre goes away, your body has *not* gotten rid of the syphilis. The only thing that can get rid of syphilis is medication.

Once the chancre(s) go away, syphilis goes into what is called the Secondary Stage. In this stage, the infected person develops a rash on their body. Most commonly this rash will show up on your hands or feet, but it could show up anywhere. Now remember, often this rash is happening without another symptom. Typically, when humans think of rashes, they think of an allergic reaction to something, like soap, for example. It might not cross someone's mind that this is related to that little bump on their penis from a couple of months ago, you know?

Some other symptoms in the Secondary Stage that may or may not happen at the same time as the rash are more flu-like in nature. Upset stomach, low-grade fever, exhaustion, sore throat, swollen glands, headache and muscle aches are all possible. Again, these symptoms are easily confused with the flu or a cold. Especially since these types of symptoms can last two to six weeks. Just like the Primary Stage, these symptoms will go away without treatment, but, just like with the Primary Stage, the syphilis is still present and can be given to another person. In fact, a person can stay in the first or second stage of this infection for months or even years. Meaning, they may not have any other additional symptoms until the infection moves into the Late Stage.

The Late Stage is the final stage for syphilis. This is a really dangerous stage for the person who has syphilis. People in this stage may develop tumors or become blind. Syphilis has also been known to damage a person's nervous system (brain) or other organs. People can actually die from untreated syphilis. The good news is that a person can get rid of syphilis with antibiotics. They can get rid of it any point, but if there has been damage done to a person's body, like if their nervous system has suffered because of the disease, the antibiotics don't eliminate that damage. Make sense? Another example would be if a person has gone blind because of syphilis and then they take antibiotics—they will get rid of the syphilis, but they will still be blind. Again, the only way you will know for sure if you have syphilis is to get tested. If you think you see a chancre, get it checked out. Weird, unknown rash? Get it checked out. Oh, and what do I mean by getting checked out? I mean see a medical provider.

Remember, you don't have to wait until you have symptoms of syphilis or any of the bacterial STIs. You can, and should, incorporate regular STI testing into your health care regimen. What's regular testing look like? It's different for each person. Some people get tested before every new partner. Some people do it every three or six months. Some people get tested annually. If you aren't sure how often you should get tested, ask your doctor!

VIRAL STIS
Things to keep in mind about viral STIs:

- Once you get a viral STI, you have it for the rest of your life.

- While you can't get rid of the virus, you can treat the symptoms.

- Some viral STIs have vaccines and others have pro-phylactic (preventative) medication.

- The only people who can diagnose viral STIs are medical professionals.

- This kind of STI can be passed from one person to another through sexual contact, exchanging fluids, and through exposure to blood and breast milk.

Genital Warts and HPV

Genital warts are commonly caused by a virus called HPV. There are many different strains of HPV and only a few of them actually lead to the growth of genital warts. So, you can have HPV and not get genital warts. And you can still have the strain of HPV that is responsible for a body grow-ing genital warts, even if you don't have any genital warts. Confused yet? Of all the STIs out there, understanding HPV is one of the most challenging.

First of all, HPV is super common. And, a lot of the time, any symptoms of HPV, like genital warts, often go away without treatment. There are some strains of HPV that can lead to increased cancer risk (cervical cancer or penile can-cer), while other strains of HPV are categorized as low-risk because all they do is cause some warts to grow on your genitalia.

HPV is pretty common. During 2013–2014, 45.2% of adults aged eighteen to fifty-nine reported having HPV. Rates were higher in people who identify as non-Hispanic black. [22] HPV is so common because it is easily transmitted through things like genital-to-genital contact even without fluids be-ing present. So, things that protect against other STIs, like condoms and dental dams, may not protect you from HPV if the warts aren't covered up. Furthermore, just because they are called genital warts doesn't mean you can't get them on other parts of your body if those other parts of the body come into contact with the wart. So, if you're performing oral sex on a penis that has genital warts, it's possible that you then can develop the warts on or in your mouth.

So how do you know if you have genital warts? Well, like I said, you might not ever actually get a wart. Or, the warts might develop inside the body and, because they are painless, you might never know you have them. But the best way to know if you have genital warts is to get tested.

---

22 "National Center for Health Statistics." Centers for Disease Control and Prevention. April 06, 2017. Accessed January 17, 2018. http://www.cdc.gov/nchs/products/databriefs/db280.htm.

You will have a better chance of a proper diagnosis if you get tested when you see an actual wart present. A wart is the same color as your skin or maybe a little more white in color. They are kind of bumpy, and a lot of people say they look like a tiny head of cauliflower. Sometimes people just get one wart, but they can also present in a cluster (so, several warts together). Just because you might have a bump on your skin, this does not mean you have genital warts, so don't freak! The only way to know for sure is to have a medical professional look at it.

If you're exposed to a genital wart, you don't immediately get a genital wart. In fact, for some people it can take months or even years for an actual wart to appear. This is one reason why HPV is so common. The most common symptom, a wart, can take a really long time to show up, but in all that time you can still transmit it to someone else. So many people can't pinpoint who exactly exposed them to the virus and, if you don't know you were exposed, you may not take the necessary precautions to keep your partner from getting exposed.

If you think you have genital warts, you will want to see a medical professional to make sure you get a proper diagnosis. A medical professional may suggest treatment for the genital warts (like freezing them or burning them—a very simple procedure done in a medical office), they might prescribe some medicine to put on them, or they may just suggest leaving them alone.

Since genital warts are caused by a strain of HPV, you can actually get a vaccination against HPV that can help your body prevent the transmission of HPV. This is the best way to prevent transmission. A person can get the HPV vaccine at any point in their life, but if a person already has HPV, the vaccine isn't going to help them. It's best to get the vaccine before becoming sexually active. Experts suggest getting the HPV vaccine in middle school (around the age of eleven or twelve).[23] The HPV vaccine is a series of shots given over several months (I know, no one likes shots, but it's better to be protected than not protected. I mean, if you can prevent getting a kind of cancer, why wouldn't you?). A person needs to get all the shots in order to be fully protected.

Hepatitis B

Hepatitis B is a viral infection that attacks the liver. It's sometimes called HBV and it can be pretty serious. Hepatitis B is really contagious. Again, it's present in fluids that are exchanged during sex (pre-ejaculate, ejaculate, and vaginal fluids). It is also present in blood and urine. Besides being at risk for transmission through sexual activity, hepatitis B can be transmitted in other ways like sharing needles (for drugs, piercings, or tattoos) or even sharing a razor or toothbrush. Sometimes a person cuts themselves when they are shaving or gets small cuts in their gums when they brush their teeth—it's the blood that is worrisome, not the saliva or skin. Hepatitis B can also be passed to a baby when it's born if the mom has it. You *can't* get hep B through kissing or sharing food, or from someone who has it coughing on you.

---

23   "HPV Vaccine for Preteens and Teens." Centers for Disease Control and Prevention. www.cdc.gov/vaccines/parents/diseases/teen/hpv.html

There are three kinds of hepatitis out there: hepatitis A, B, and C. And all of these affect the liver. You can actually get a vaccine for two of these kinds of hepatitis: A and B. There is not currently a vaccine for hepatitis C. It's recommended that children receive the hepatitis A vaccine after their first birthday. For adults who haven't received the vaccine, it's recommended for those traveling to countries with high rates of hepatitis A. We are only talking about hepatitis B in this book because it's the only form of hepatitis that can be transmitted through sexual activity. [24]

Like many other STIs, hepatitis B often doesn't have symptoms. When someone does have symptoms, they are really similar to symptoms of the flu or a bad cold, so it's hard for people to pinpoint exactly what is going on. If you get hepatitis B, the symptoms usually appear anywhere between six weeks to six months later. Just like the flu, the symptoms can stick around for a few weeks and then go away. Generally, the symptoms include a fever, feeling sick to the stomach, a headache, joint pain and fatigue. Because hep B affects the liver, a person can also have dark urine (pee), whitish poop, and yellowish-colored skin (jaundice).

The best way to prevent getting hepatitis B is to get vaccinated against it. You should get the vaccine before becoming sexually active. Just like with the HPV vaccine, the hepatitis B vaccine is a series of three shots (again, you're going to have to get over the shot thing, because well, hepatitis B is really contagious and why not protect yourself? You kinda need your liver in order to live a healthy life). Even if you're

---

24 "Hepatitis A - in Short." Centers for Disease Control and Prevention. Accessed July 13, 2018. https://www.cdc.gov/vaccines/vpd/hepa/public/in-short-adult.html#who

vaccinated against hepatitis B, you're still going to want to protect yourself and your partner by using condoms.

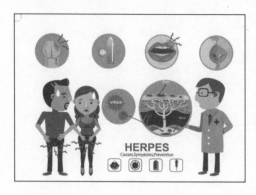

Herpes

Herpes is another fairly common STI. Approximately one in six people aged fourteen to forty-nine in the United States has herpes.[25]

Herpes is caused by two different viruses: herpes simplex virus type 1 (HSV-1) and herpes simplex virus type 2 (HSV-2). Pretty creative names, huh? While it's interesting to know that herpes is caused by two different strains, that doesn't affect how the virus shows up in your body (that is, if it even shows symptoms. Did you know that 90% of all those people don't even know they have herpes?).[26]

Since people who have herpes often don't show symptoms, it can be pretty hard to diagnose unless you get an STI test and therefore, it gets spread pretty easily – especially since it can be spread through skin-to-skin contact. That includes oral, anal, and vaginal sex, and even kissing. Without testing, the only way you will know if you have herpes is by the presence of sores. Typically, these sores

25 "Genital Herpes - CDC Fact Sheet." Centers for Disease Control and Prevention. Accessed July 11, 2018. https://www.cdc.gov/std/herpes/stdfact-herpes.htm
26 Bradley H. Markowitz LE, Gibson T, McQuillan GM. Seroprevalence of herpes simplex virus types 1 and 2 – United States, 1999-2010. J Infect Dis. 2014 Feb 1;209(3):325-33.

are pretty painful. They are usually round in shape and are open wounds. They can also present as blisters, and besides being painful they can be itchy too. Since herpes is so contagious, they can show up wherever contact has happened. They can be on the genitals, anus, inside the vagina, on the mouth and lips and even in your throat. If you touch a sore with your finger and touch another part of the body where the fluids from the sore can enter the body, you can transmit the virus (yeah, it's that contagious). And sometimes these sores can be mistaken for something else. If someone doesn't know that the sore is actually a herpes sore, they might not be as careful as they should be and this can lead to unnecessary transmission.

There isn't a cure for herpes. So, once you get it, you have it for life and you can transmit it to another person. Even if you don't see sores on a person's body, they can still have herpes and transmit it to another person. Even though herpes is very contagious, it can't live for very long on the outside of the body if there isn't an open sore present. (An open sore will often be wet with pus and that pus contains the virus.) Activities like hugging and holding hands are pretty safe.

If you get herpes, it's almost impossible to determine who you got it from. Herpes can lay dormant in your nervous system for months and even years before showing up. Herpes outbreaks will typically happen in the same place on the body over and over again and they are especially common when a person's immune system is weak (like when they are sick or under a lot of stress). Some people get one herpes sore their whole life and then never have another one. Some people get outbreaks all the time. Some people never have an outbreak. Everyone presents a little differently.

While you can't get rid of the herpes virus, you can treat the actual sores with medication. Some types of herpes sores can be treated with over-the-counter medication while others will need a prescription. There are even medications that can help people suppress a herpes outbreak. But remember, just because you can't see a herpes sore doesn't mean you can't transmit the virus to someone else or get it from someone. You can't tell someone has herpes just by looking at them.

Because herpes is so hard to diagnose, it's important to get checked out by a medical professional as soon as you see a sore. Your health care provider will have an easier time diagnosing whether you have herpes or not if you have an actual sore present, because they can swab the sore and take a sample of the pus (fluid) for analysis. If you see a health care provider and don't have an open sore, they can test for the virus by taking a blood sample.

Remember, since the herpes viruses are so contagious, pretty much everyone carries one strain or another. There are lots of different kinds of herpes viruses out there and they present differently in different people. Take as many precautions as you can to protect yourself from getting it, but don't freak out if you get it. Remember, herpes can even be spread through behaviors besides sexual ones.

HIV and AIDS

HIV or Human Immunodeficiency Virus is a serious viral infection that breaks down a person's immune system. The immune system is what helps humans fight infections and keeps people healthy. If someone's immune system is weakened, a person can get really sick and even die from an infection or disease that could normally be defeated. There are approximately 1.1 million people in the United States living with HIV.[27]

HIV is spread through fluids that are exchanged in sex: pre-ejaculate, ejaculate, and vaginal fluids. HIV is also spread through blood. So, it can be spread through non-sexual acts like sharing needles. HIV can also be spread to a baby through the ingestion of breast milk. HIV enters the body through mucous membranes as well as cuts and sores—even when these cuts are super-duper tiny, like small, almost microscopic abrasions. These abrasions can be caused by normal sexual activity and you may not even notice that they are there. They can be on a penis, inside the vagina, or in the anus. You can't get HIV from kissing, sharing utensils with an infected person, holding hands, hugging, coughing, or using the same toilet seat as someone who is HIV positive (meaning they have tested positive on an HIV test). It is extremely unlikely to get HIV from a blood transfusion. In fact, the risk is 1 in 1.5 million.[28]

Once a person gets HIV, the virus will stay in their body forever because there isn't a cure. However, there are medications that can help people fight the effects of the virus in the body as well as help prevent its spread to partners. Without treatment, though, people will almost always die. Don't mess around with knowing your HIV status. Get tested.

HIV and AIDS, although often used interchangeably, are not the same thing. AIDS stands for Acquired Immune Deficiency Syndrome. AIDS is a disease caused by HIV (the virus) and a person who has HIV does not always get

27 "HIV in the United States: At a Glance." Centers for Disease Control and Prevention. Accessed July 11, 2018. https://www.cdc.gov/hiv/statistics/overview/ataglance.html
28 "HIV Transmission Through Transfusion." Centers for Disease Control and Prevention. Accessed July 11, 2017. https://www.cdc.gov/mmwr/preview/mmwrhtml/mm5941a3.htm.

AIDS. When a person gets AIDS, any infection can be really dangerous. Having AIDS is the most dangerous stage of HIV. Without treatment, a person typically develops AIDS after ten years of having HIV.[29]

The symptoms of HIV and then AIDS change over time and depend on whether or not a person is being treated. When a person is first exposed to HIV, they probably don't know. It's pretty common for a person to feel healthy for a long time. Some people don't show any symptoms of HIV for up to ten years after infection. That's a long time to live with a potentially deadly virus! (Just another reason to get regularly tested.)

When a person is first exposed they may feel flu-like symptoms: fever, achy, upset stomach, headache. Not only are these symptoms like so many other STIs, they are like many other illnesses. If you experience these types of symptoms after having unprotected sex or sharing needles, you're going to want to stop having sex and get tested. You want to stop having sex because this is the time when HIV is going to be the most contagious in your body and you're most likely to spread it to another partner. Getting tested is the only way you can know for sure whether the symptoms you're having are just a normal flu, or whether they are related to HIV. The flu-like symptoms will eventually go away. But just because they go away doesn't mean that you aren't able to spread the virus to other people. Whether you are showing symptoms or not, you're still carrying the virus and can still give it to another person if you're sharing needles or having unprotected sex.

After the beginning symptoms of HIV go away, the virus is still damaging your body. HIV kills cells in your immune

29 "Official Site." Planned Parenthood. Accessed January 17, 2018. http://www.plannedparenthood.org/.

system. These cells are commonly called "T cells." When your T cells are killed, the count of T cells in the body goes down. The lower the count, the easier it is for the body to become sick. As in, sicknesses that would normally take you out for a few days can become life-threatening.

A person may develop AIDS after living with HIV for a long time, because the disease has taken a toll on the body. Typically, this is about ten years after exposure to the virus. Symptoms of AIDS include:

- Thrush (a thick, white coating on the tongue)
- Sore throat
- Chronic yeast infections and pelvic inflammatory disease for those who are female-bodied
- Dizziness and vertigo
- Headaches
- Extreme unexplained weight loss
- Coughing and shortness of breath
- Fever
- Unexplained bleeding (especially in the mouth, nose, anus, or vagina)
- Bruising
- Unexplained rashes and skin legions
- Losing feeling in your hands and feet or losing coordination

Again, these symptoms alone could be caused by many things. But if you have tested positive for HIV, they could be the symptoms signifying that the HIV has gone into a more progressed state of AIDS.

It's important to remember that millions of people are living normal lives despite their diagnosis. Testing positive for HIV is *not* a death sentence. In fact, there are many medical breakthroughs that are helping to improve the quality of life for those with HIV. Anti-retroviral therapy, or ART, can slow down the effects of the disease on the body. But the sooner a person starts taking the medication the better it will be for the body. Because an HIV diagnosis can be hard to hear, there are many resources available to help. HIV.gov is a great place to go to understand treatment options as well as find mental health assistance and advice on how best to talk with your family and friends about your diagnosis. There is still a lot of misinformation out there about HIV and what a positive diagnosis means.

While preventing HIV looks really similar to preventing any STI (use a condom or dental dam for sexual acts, participate in no-risk behaviors like masturbation, kissing, and dry-humping), it's important to remember that it's easier for a person to get HIV from another person if they have open sores or cuts that fluids can get into. There is no vaccine available for HIV but some people who are at extreme risk for HIV (like IV drug users or people whose partners have a positive diagnosis) can take PrEP. PrEP stands for "pre-exposure prophylaxis"—a medication that can help prevent a person from getting HIV. It's very effective but is not a guarantee that the person won't get HIV. A medical professional can help you to figure out if PrEP is something that would be good for you to be on.

If you think it's possible you have been exposed to HIV, there is also PEP. That stands for "post-exposure prophylaxis." By taking PEP, a person can reduce their chance of contracting HIV even if they have been exposed to it. Again, it's not guaranteed but has shown to be helpful for many people. A medical professional can help you determine if this type of treatment is something that would help you as it depends on the situation (like when you might have been exposed).

STI's: Wrap "It" Up

Just remember, unless you have medical training, you can't diagnose yourself or a friend. If you notice something different going on (like increased discharge if you're female-bodied or any discharge if you're male-bodied), or you have engaged in unprotected sexual activity, go get tested. It's easy and fast. If you have an STI and leave it untreated, it can become a bigger problem later on.

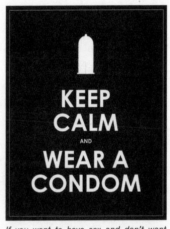

If you want to have sex and don't want an STI? Simple. Use a condom or dental dam to make sure you and your partner are protected.

STIs like gonorrhea, chlamydia, and syphilis can even lead to infertility (or the inability to have children) if they aren't treated in a timely manner. Also, if you don't know you have an STI, you might pass it on to another person without even knowing it. So, get tested often (at least once a year or before a new partner) to make sure you and your partner are safe and healthy. And make sure you ask your partner (and your partner asks you) whether they know their STI status. Just remember that getting STI testing is a normal part of your medical care and nothing to be embarrassed about.

Some people feel like having an STI is something to be ashamed of or that it means a person is dirty, or that they have lots of sex with different people. In reality, half of the people in the U.S. will get an STI in their lifetime, and people fifteen to twenty-four-years-old are the most likely to get STIs.[30] That's a lot of people. So, it's really common and, by empowering yourself to know your STI status, you can actually help make sure STI testing and communication about STIs are normalized. You can be a part of helping rates of STIs go down!

Also, if you get an STI, this doesn't mean you can't have a perfectly healthy and happy sex life or have a romantic relationship. Millions of people have an STI (or several STIs) and have great relationships and sexually fulfilling lives. Of course, being diagnosed with an STI is no fun. But, lots of STIs are curable, and those that aren't can still be treated. Having an STI is nothing to be ashamed of. But it does mean that when you're having sexual relationships, you need to be up front and honest with your partner to keep both of you safe.

Having a conversation about your STI isn't always easy. People worry about being judged. They fear that telling a partner might change their opinion of them, whether or not their partner wants to be sexually active with them. Here's the thing, though. You care about this person, right? Enough to have sex or engage in sexual activity with them? You have respect for them? Sharing your STI status is a part of showing respect for your partner. It's helping your partner to make

---

30 Centers for Disease Control and Prevention. Sexually Transmitted Diseases in the United States, 2008

a consensual decision with all of the information. Remember these hints when you're disclosing your STI status: [31]

- Keep calm. Millions of people have STIs, and for most couples, STI status isn't insurmountable. Go into the conversation with a calm and positive attitude. Having an STI is a health issue. That's it. It doesn't mean anything about who you are.

- Make it a two-way convo. Remember that STIs are *super* common. Who's to say your partner doesn't have something they need to tell you about their STI status? Remember, you should be talking about this *before* you become sexually active. A great way to establish trust and show the two of you respect each other. Before you start being sexually intimate, go get tested. Together, with friends, whatever. Just *go*.

- Know the facts. There are so many myths out there about STIs. Don't get caught up in the misinformation! While the internet has a lot of great info out there, make sure you're getting your information from a reputable site like www.cdc.gov or www.planned-parenthood.org. And whatever you do, do *not* search for images of the disease on the internet. Trust me on this one. First of all, there are a lot of mislabeled pictures, but those pictures that are there are like, the *worst* cases ever recorded. The pictures are nothing like most people's experiences with STIs. Also, know how to protect yourself and your partner. Know what sexual activities are especially risky for the STI you

31 "Official Site." Planned Parenthood. Accessed January 17, 2018. http://www.plannedparenthood.org/.

have (or are trying to avoid) and steer clear of those activities. Or make sure you're being especially cautious and using proper protection.

- Think about when and where. Having this conversation is serious. You're going to want to make sure you're in a head space where you feel comfortable having it, and that neither you or your partner is distracted by the latest music video or by homework. It might sound lame, but it also doesn't hurt to practice what you want to say. What about using your parents as a sounding board? They might be able to give you a few pointers. Maybe they've even had this conversation before and have some ideas of what is helpful to know, say, or do.

- Make sure you're safe. If you are worried your partner might try to hurt you or that having this conversation could be dangerous, take precautions to keep yourself safe. Maybe you're in a public place like a park where you can have some privacy but other people are around. Or maybe you talk on the phone or send an email. Remember, if you're concerned about a partner being abusive, there is help. Talk to your friends, talk to your parents, or you can even call the National Domestic Violence Hotline at 1-800-799-SAFE.

WHAT IS IT LIKE TO GET AN STI TEST?

Many people don't get tested because they are scared or embarrassed. But, as you have read, STIs are very common. And the only way to know for sure if you have one is to get tested. If you're female-bodied, it's important to know that STI testing is not part of an annual exam. STI testing is also not part of an annual physical. If you want to be tested for STIs, you have to advocate for it and request testing from your doctor.

Getting tested isn't scary and it's really important. Let's break it down so you know what you are getting into and feel comfortable with this really important responsibility. First, it's important to know that different health clinics test differently. Health care providers that specialize in sexual health care, like a Planned Parenthood, may go further in-depth with you than another health care provider (like a pediatrician, for example) because that's what they do—care for your sexual health. While someone who is a general health care provider may have a slightly different protocol. Here's a cheat sheet of what a health care provider will do to assess your STI risk (regardless of where you're seeking testing):

- Visual inspection: if you have sores or bumps, someone will need to look at them to see if they are signs of an infection

- Urine sample (peeing in a cup)

- Blood sample (drawing blood with a needle or with a finger prick)

- Tissue sample (using a cotton swab, the inside of the mouth or genitals is swiped)

A doctor or nurse is also going to ask you questions about your sexual behavior. It's important for you to be honest with the doctor or nurse so they can properly treat you. They are going to ask you about the kind(s) of sex you have (like whether it's oral, anal or vaginal) and they are going to ask you about how many sexual partners you have had.

They will also ask who you have sex with (whether male- or female-bodied) and whether you use protection like a condom or dental dam. Answering these types of questions might feel embarrassing, but the doctor or nurse needs to know the truth so they can help you, and they won't be able to help you if you don't give them all the information they need.

Sometimes the results of a positive STI test are reported to the county or state health department. This varies from state to state. Some states have an anonymous reporting structure while others have a confidential structure. The reason positive test results are reported to the health departments is that STIs are considered a public health concern. By tracking those who test positive, infection trends can be identified. Once identified, the proper community health programs can be implemented to try to eliminate the disease. It's the intent of the public health departments to eliminate any diseases that they can. Take polio, for example. Due to the efforts of the public health departments, polio has been all but eradicated from the U.S. It's the hope that similar interventions can do the same for STIs. In fact, it has been through the tracking, education, and funding of the public health departments that vaccines have been developed and made available for some STIs and that transmission rates for STIs have decreased.

CONVERSATION STARTERS . . .

• • • • • • • • • • •

The conversation starters are designed to be prompts for having conversations. Feel free to use them in the way that feels right to you.

Talking about STIs can be hard. Not only is it hard to talk with a medical provider about what is going on, it's hard to talk to your parents and partner about what is going on. Fear of being judged or having a difficult conversation can be non-starters for people. But these conversations are critical to your ability to stay healthy. Here are some ideas of things teens can ask their parents to help feel more comfortable.

Questions for Teens to Ask Their Parents

- Have you ever gotten an STI test? Why or why not?

- Have you ever known anyone with an STI? Who was it? How did you find out?

- Have you ever talked to a doctor or nurse about your sexual history? Why or why not? If you did, what was it like?

Questions for Parents to Ask Their Teens

- Have you ever gotten an STI test?

- Do you need help setting up an STI test?

- How do you plan on keeping yourself safe from STIs?

- When you have sex, or are going to have sex, what are some things you talk to your partner about to make sure you aren't at risk for STIs?

14

CONTRACEPTION:
THE LOW DOWN

We've already discussed low risk to high risk and talked about STIs, but what if you or your partner are at risk for pregnancy? As we've already talked about, the only sure way you won't get pregnant or get someone pregnant is to not have vaginal sex. If you're ready to have sex or engage in sexual behaviors and want to minimize the risk of pregnancy, you're going to want to use contraception.

The good news? In 2011, the teen pregnancy rate hit a record low of fifty-two pregnancies per one thousand women aged fifteen to nineteen! That means that when teens are having sex where the penis is going into the vagina, they are using more effective forms of contraception. It also means that if teens are having penis-to-vagina sex, they are still at risk for becoming pregnant. [32]

32 Kost K and Maddow-Zimet I, U.S. Teenage Pregnancies, Births and Abortions, 2011: National Trends by Age, Race and Ethnicity, New York: Guttmacher Institute, 2016.

In order to pick the most effective contraception for you or your partner, keep these things in mind:

- How comfortable am I with my body?

- Is this something I can do on my own or do I need to involve my partner?

- How much does it cost? (Keep in mind lots of states and health departments, as well as private providers, have programs that can help cover the cost of the method.)

- Where can I get it?

- Do I need to go to a health care center for a procedure or prescription?

There are different forms of contraception. Some have hormones, some don't. Some you have to think about daily, while others last ten years. And some are more effective at preventing pregnancy than others. There is only one type of contraception, however, that also protects a person from STI transmission: the condom. Buckle up, peeps—this is a lot of info!

MOST EFFECTIVE FORMS OF CONTRACEPTION
Less than 1 pregnancy per 100 women in a year
Let's start by taking a look at the most effective forms of contraception: those that are permanent (meaning, they typically last a person's whole life) or those that last for years at a time without the user needing to think about them.

Sterilization

It's nearly impossible for a teenager to get a permanent form of contraception because, well, its permanent. Lots of people consider these as they become older when they know for sure that they do not want or are finished having children. It's popular because once the procedure has been completed there is little or nothing to think about with regard to preventing pregnancy.

For a male-bodied person, the permanent form of contraception is called a **vasectomy**. A male-bodied person's vas deferens (remember the anatomy from page 61?) are severed and therefore, when the male-bodied person ejaculates, the sperm can't leave the body. In some cases, a vasectomy can be reversed (again, this is going to require a small procedure) but that is not always successful. A vasectomy is not one hundred percent effective at preventing pregnancy. It's unlikely (but has happened) that a male-bodied person's vas deferens grows back together. It's more common, though, that a male-bodied person does not use adequate back-up protection after the procedure for the prescribed amount of time and there is still viable sperm living in the vas deferens for a time after the procedure. It is important for a male-bodied person who has had this procedure to protect themselves and their partner from STIs. A male-bodied person who has this procedure will still ejaculate fluid—there just won't be any sperm in the fluid.

If a female decides they want to be sterilized, they will have a few more options. These range from a complete hysterectomy (removal of the ovaries, cervix and uterus) to tubal ligation (severing of the fallopian tubes) to a less invasive surgical procedure called Essure. Essure is a newer procedure that involves the doctor inserting small metal coils into the fallopian tubes, which then cause the tubes to scar and become blocked off so the egg and sperm can't meet.

IUDs

Since sterilization isn't really an option for a teen, let's talk about some options that are available and last a really long time: Long Acting Reversible Contraception, or LARCs. These are the most effective forms of contraception available and *are* a long-term option that teens who are female-bodied can get. LARCs include IUDs, or "the implant." An IUD is an "Intrauterine Device." This is a device that is inserted inside a female-bodied person's uterus. It's made out of plastic and shaped like a "T."

At the time of publication, there are five different kinds of IUDs out there and these are broken into two categories: with hormones and without hormones. Both types of IUDs work pretty similarly. They prevent how the sperm cells move. This interference means they can't get to the egg and, if the sperm can't find the egg, pregnancy won't happen. A health care provider must insert the IUD to make sure it's properly placed inside the uterus. The proper placement contributes to its effectiveness. In order to put it in the body, the health care provider uses a special instrument that opens the cervix so that the IUD can go through. Once placed, strings attached to the IUD will come through the cervix and stay in the vagina. These strings can help the female-bodied person make sure the IUD is in the proper place and, if or when the person is ready, the strings will enable the removal of the IUD. Don't worry, the strings become soft and most partners report that they can't feel them during sexual intercourse.

What happens if I were to become pregnant on an IUD? It's possible. Usually, the pregnancy is okay, but only a doctor can say for sure. Each case is different, and a health care provider can help you to figure out what the options are for you.

A hormonal IUD has the hormone called progestin in it. This hormone naturally occurs in the female body. By adding synthetic progesterone to the body through the IUD, it helps to prevent pregnancy by thickening the cervical mucus (this is the same stuff as "discharge" that you might find in your underpants). When the mucus is super thick, it acts as a barrier and prevents the sperm from getting to the egg. Additionally, the hormones that are in the IUD can sometimes prevent your ovaries from actually releasing an egg. If there isn't an egg, a person can't get pregnant. These types of IUDs can last from three to six years.

A copper IUD can last up to 12 years and it doesn't have any hormones. The copper coil is what makes this effective at preventing pregnancy. Sperm don't like the copper and the copper basically "deactivates" the sperm, making it almost impossible for the sperm to get to the egg.

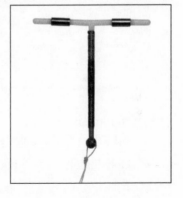

IUDs are a really great option for those who know they don't want to be pregnant now, but in a few years, or maybe just someday might want to become pregnant. When a person decides they want to become pregnant, they visit a health care provider and that provider will remove the IUD using the strings that hang out through the cervix in the vagina. Both insertion and removal are relatively painless but can cause some discomfort.

Side effects for an IUD vary per person. Some people get heavier periods, while others stop having their period altogether. It's important to discuss the side effects and what to expect with a medical professional. A medical provider can also help you figure out how to lessen those side effects.

DID YOU KNOW that an IUD can also be used as emergency contraception? It's true! If you have unprotected sex or if your birth control method fails, you can see a medical provider and have an IUD inserted within five days. This is only true for the copper IUD (ParaGard). In fact, it's the most effective form of EC as it's 99.9% effective at preventing pregnancy when it's inserted within five days of unprotected sex. Another thing that's cool about using the copper IUD as EC? It's then your regular contraception for up to 12 years after that! Pretty sweet!

Things to remember:
- An IUD is 99% effective
- Only female-bodied people can get an IUD
- IUDs do *not* prevent the transmission of STIs
- You have to go to a health care provider to get an IUD, but an IUD can last up to 12 years
- IUDs cost from $0-$1,300

The Implant

The implant, also called Nexplanon, (there is also an older version called Implanon you might have heard about) is a small, thin rod of plastic that contains hormones. It's about 1.5 inches long and is inserted into a female-bodied person's arm by a health care provider. Once it is put in the body, the user doesn't have to think about it again for four years!

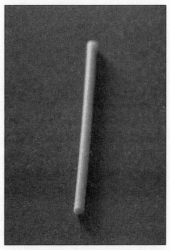

Made of plastic, the implant is flexible and designed to move with your body.

In order to get it into the arm and under the skin, the health care provider will first numb the area of insertion with a shot. Then the health care provider will make a tiny incision and insert the implant. After the numbing shot wears off, the individual won't feel the implant. They might be a little sore right after it is inserted but that will go away. (It might feel like you got pinched.)

The implant contains both estrogen and progestin. Like the hormonal IUD, the implant's hormones not only prevent the eggs from leaving the ovaries (stopping ovulation), but the hormones also thicken the cervical mucus, which makes it difficult for the sperm to get past the cervix. A super effective form of contraception, but the implant doesn't protect against STIs.

If you get an implant, it can become effective immediately as long as the individual gets the implant during the first five days of their period. If not, the individual will want to use a back-up method like a condom for the first week they have their implant.

Most people's side effects from the implant go away after a few months. For some, in the first 6–12 months, an individual may find their period becomes slightly irregular, either with a heavier flow or spotting between periods. But most people report that their periods become lighter, and a lot of people stop having their periods altogether after one year on the implant. Common side effects include headaches, breast pain or tenderness, weight gain, feeling sick to your stomach, and cysts on your ovaries. More serious complications from the implant can happen with regards to the incision or point of entry for the implant. If an individual chooses this method of contraception, they will need to make sure they are comfortable caring for the incision.

Ovarian cysts are small growths on or in the ovary that may be made of solid material or filled with fluid (called pus). Many female-bodied people never even know when they have a cyst because they can't feel them and they can go away on their own, but sometimes cysts can make you feel uncomfortable or become painful. The pain might feel sharp or it could be less noticeable. It usually comes and goes. If you have any of these symptoms, you should talk to your health care provider. They can do an exam, which might include a vaginal ultrasound. Unlike an ultrasound that a female-bodied person may have when they are visibly pregnant, which is when a health care provider puts lubrication over the abdomen and swipes an instrument over the uterus, a vaginal ultrasound is done by inserting a lubricated medical instrument that kind of looks like a microphone into the vagina. A vaginal ultrasound allows the doctor to see inside your body.

After four years, or if the female-bodied person wants to become pregnant or change their contraception method at any point while using the implant, they need to see a health care provider to get the implant removed from their arm. The removal of the implant is similar to the insertion. The arm is numbed with a shot (remember that pinch from insertion? It's just like that). The doctor or nurse will then make a very small incision and use a tool to remove the implant. Again, the arm might be sore as it heals, but after the implant is out, your body will go back to "normal," which means that you can also get pregnant as soon as it's removed if you don't use contraception.

Things to remember:

- The implant is 99% effective
- Only female-bodied people can get the implant
- The implant does not prevent the transmission of STIs
- You have to go to a health care provider to get the implant every four years
- Costs $0-$1,300

LESS EFFECTIVE FORMS OF CONTRACEPTION
Out of 100 Female-Bodied People, 6–12 Will Become Pregnant On These Methods of Contraception

Don't get me wrong, these forms of contraception are really solid. In fact, the contraception methods that fall in this category are some of the most popular and have been around for a long time. This category consists of hormonal methods that must be prescribed and one form that has to be fit by a health care provider. No matter what, you're heading into a health care provider to access these types of contraception.

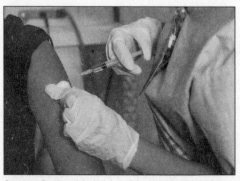

Caption: Getting the shot is quick and relatively painless. It's always given to you by a medical professional in a clinic or doctor's office.

The Shot

The birth control shot, or Depo Provera (Depo), is an injectable contraception method. The shot contains the hormone progestin which is similar to the progestin produced in the body. The extra progestin prevents a female-bodied person from ovulating or releasing an egg. Remember: no egg, no pregnancy. It also thickens the cervical mucus which provides a barrier for the sperm. The shot doesn't protect against STI transmission.

Because the shot is, well, a shot, you need to go to your health care provider to get it. The good news? You only go every 12–13 weeks. The bad news? You're going to need an appointment so make sure you schedule the appointments in a way that is going to work for you. If you know transportation is a problem, or you don't have easy access to a provider, the shot isn't going to be a good option for you. The biggest challenge with ensuring the shot prevents against pregnancy is user error. Meaning, if you miss a shot or are late getting it (because life happens!), you're not going to be protected against pregnancy until you get the shot again and have followed the recommended amount of time until it becomes effective. Until you know it's effective you should use a back-up method like a condom. If you're already sexually active before you get the shot, a health care provider will give you a pregnancy test to make sure you aren't pregnant before they give the injection. Similarly, if you're late in getting your next shot or you skip a dose, they will test you to see if you're pregnant, just to make sure.

As with other medication, there are side effects to the shot. Possible side effects include your period stopping, bleeding for longer than usual during your period, or spotting between periods. Some people also report that they feel sick to their stomachs (nauseous), have headaches, gain weight, and/or have breast tenderness. But, if you get the shot and decide you don't like it, no problem! The hormones will level out after three months and you can try something different.

Things to remember:

- Because people can make mistakes when using the shot, the typical effectiveness is 94%

- Only female-bodied people can get the shot

- The shot does not prevent the transmission of STIs

- You have to go to a health care provider to get the shot every 12–13 weeks
- Costs $0-$100 per shot

The Pill

The birth control pill, or "pill," has been around for a long time. It was the first form of hormonal contraception. Since it has been around a long time, manufac-

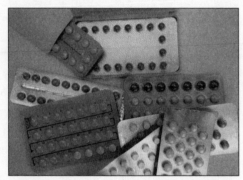

There are so many different kinds of pills out there. Each kind has a different dosage and combination of hormones but they are all designed to prevent pregnancy.

turers have made many different kinds. Not only are there lots of brands of pills out there, but there are lots of different doses. Just like the shot, the pill is made up of hormones. Some pills are made up of just progestin, but the majority of pills out there have various combinations of both progestin and estrogen. Since everybody is different, every body produces hormones differently. Meaning, everyone's hormone balance looks different. They are all effective in preventing pregnancy when used consistently and correctly (more on that in a few), but have, depending on the person taking them, different side effects. If you decide to start taking the pill, you will want to give your body 2–3 months to get used to the hormones. Many female-bodied people find that the side effects go away. But, sometimes, a female-bodied person has to try out a couple different kinds of pills to find the right mix that works for them with the fewest side effects. Some side effects from pills are: moodiness, acne, heavy periods, weight gain, spotting between periods, or not having a period at all. If someone is interested in using the pill but experiences unpleasant side effects, they should see their health care provider to see if there is a better fit. Until the female-bodied person figures out the right combo they should use a back-up method like a condom.

Endometriosis is when a female-bodied person has uterine tissue growing outside the uterus, typically in the pelvis (on the uterus, fallopian tubes, and/or ovaries). It can also grow on the bladder or intestines. Endometriosis can affect a female-bodied person of any age who is menstruating. Female-bodied people who have endometriosis have different experiences with it. It typically presents with painful cramping during different times of the menstrual cycle, but especially during the period. The pain can be very debilitating for some and disrupt their day-to-day activities. But some female-bodied individuals aren't bothered by severe symptoms. Each body is different. If you're having extremely uncomfortable periods and/or cramping in your pelvic area, you should talk to a health care provider. There are several different options available to help manage the discomfort or even eliminate it.[33]

33 "Endometriosis Foundation of America." Endometriosis : Causes - Symptoms - Diagnosis - and Treatment. January 16, 2018. Accessed January 17, 2018. http://www.endofound.org/.

The pill is pretty easy to use. You simply swallow a pill. The hard part is remembering to do it! Remember above where we talked about using it consistently and correctly? This is where that's important. The user wants to take the pill at approximately the same time every day. If you're the type of person that needs a reminder, there are lots of apps out there that help female-bodied people track their periods and remind them to take their pills. You can also set a reminder on your phone. If you forget to take a pill, you want to take it as soon as you remember. Depending on how long it's been, you might want to use a back-up method like a condom.

The most common pack of pills lasts 28 days and is called a 28-day pack. If this is the contraception you choose, you would take 1 pill with hormones in it every day for the first 21 days. The last 7 pills in the 28-day pack are placebo pills, to be taken during the last week of your cycle. (They don't have any hormones in them; you take them to make sure you stay on schedule.) Typically, a female-bodied person will get their period while they are taking these placebo pills. The pill is great for regulating a person's period. Don't worry: even though you're technically not getting hormones during that week, you are still protected from getting pregnant.

The pill can also come in 21-day packs and even 91-day packs. 21-day packs work just like the 28-day packs, there just aren't any placebos and the person on this type of pill will need to remember to start the pill again after being off the pill for one week. As for the 91-day packs, these are designed for the individual to take 12 weeks' worth of hormone pills in a row. After 12 weeks, there is one week of placebo pills where a female-bodied person will have their period.

Some people who don't do well on a pill that contains both estrogen and progestin (because they have bad side effects or a pre-existing condition like migraines) can take a pill with just progestin and still enjoy the ease of taking a pill. Progestin-only pills only come in the 28-day pack option at the time of publication. Side effects for these pills look a little different than the combination pills.

> If skipping your period seems like a good option for you, you don't have to be on the 91-day pack, but you should talk to your health care provider for further guidance.

Things to remember:

- When the pill is used consistently and correctly, it can be 99% effective at preventing pregnancy. However, using the pill flawlessly isn't always what happens. Because people can make mistakes when using the pill, the typical effectiveness is 91%.

- Only female-bodied people can take the pill

- The pill does not prevent the transmission of STIs

- You have to have a prescription for the pill

- Pills range in cost from $0-$50

> Did you know that it is commonly believed that the efficacy of the birth control pill is affected by antibiotics? It actually depends on the antibiotic. If you are prescribed an antibiotic and you are on birth control pills, be sure to talk to your health care provider about whether it will lower the efficacy of the pill (and make the pill less effective at preventing pregnancy).

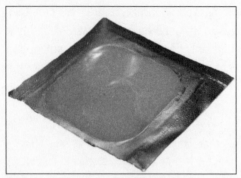

Caption: The Patch feels a lot like a thick band aid. Unfortunately, it only comes in one color.

The Patch

Another hormonal method that is just as effective as the pill when used consistently and correctly is "the patch." The patch is like a sticker (only really strong with lots of adhesive) that a female-bodied person wears either on their upper stomach area, upper arm, butt, or back. It contains hormones and looks a lot like a square Band-Aid. An individual wears the patch for three weeks and then doesn't wear one for one week (which is the week they have their period). Patches must be changed every seven days. So the user should wear three patches in a row and then take one week off.

Similar to other forms of hormonal contraception, the patch contains both estrogen and progestin which are absorbed through your skin into your body. Also, like other hormonal methods, the patch prevents ovulation, or the releasing of an egg from the ovary, and thickens the cervical mucus so a sperm can't get by. Like other hormonal methods, the patch doesn't prevent the transmission of STIs.

As with other hormonal methods, the patch is prescribed by a health care provider. However, you can get many "doses" of the patch at once to reduce the amount of times you need to go to a pharmacy or clinic. Also, you put the patch on your own body (or if you want to wear it on your back you will need the help of a parent, friend or partner). Since you leave each patch on your body for one week until it needs to be changed, this form of contraception has less to remember, but the user is still going to want to mark their calendar or set a reminder on their phone so they can keep track of how long the patch has been on the body and remember when to change it, as well as remember the week that they don't wear a patch at all. In order to make the patch the most effective, you want to change it roughly at the same time of day each time. You don't want to wear a patch longer than the one-week time period. When you first start using the patch, you will want to use a back-up method, like a condom, for the first seven days. After those first days of consistent and correct use, you're protected from pregnancy!

Other than how long you wear the patch, consistent and correct use has to do with how and where on the body the patch is applied. Make sure it's put on the parts of the body we have already discussed. Applying the patch is relatively easy. The thing you will want to remember is to not put lotion or oil on the skin before applying the patch as this will reduce the stickiness. It's also suggested that you put the patch in a different place than the one before it to reduce the chance that your skin becomes irritated by the adhesive. Just like a Band-Aid, to apply the patch you peel off the plastic back, which reveals the sticky side. You put the sticky side on dry, clean skin and press down for roughly 10 seconds. Other than regularly checking to make sure it's sticking properly, you shouldn't have to think about it more than once a week when it's time to change it. You can shower, swim, and participate in normal activities—no problem.

It is possible that the patch might become loose (like

the corners lifting up) or even fall off. This doesn't happen often, but it can happen. Don't worry! According to Planned Parenthood, here's what to do:

"If the patch got loose or fell off and it has been less than two days, put the patch back on. If it won't stick, or you don't have it, put on a new patch right away. Your patch change day will stay the same. You'll still be protected from pregnancy.

"If the patch got loose or fell off and it has been more than two days (or you don't know how long it's been off), start a new, four-week cycle by putting on a new patch right away. This is your new patch change day from now on. For the next seven days, use a condom or female condom to prevent pregnancy if you have vaginal sex."[34]

When it comes time to change your patch, you will want to make sure you dispose of it safely—put it in a plastic bag or wrap it in toilet paper so it doesn't stick to anyone and a pet can't get to it. Never flush a patch down a toilet! Some other things to keep in mind about the use of a patch: keep them in a safe place that is at room temperature (not too hot and not too cold). Keep the package that it comes in sealed until you're ready to use it. Once the package is opened, you need to use it ASAP. If you forget to change it on the scheduled day, you're going to have to start over. Sorry! Put on a new patch as soon as you remember and then this is going to be your new start date. Don't forget that back-up method of protection for seven days (like a condom)!

As with other forms of hormonal contraception, the user can experience some side effects. These will usually go away within two to three months of use. The side effects are similar to what we've already talked about too: feeling sick to your

---

34 "Official Site." Planned Parenthood. Accessed January 17, 2018. http://www.plannedparenthood.org/.

MAKING SENSE OF "IT"

stomach, tender breasts, a change in your period and/or spotting between periods. Another side effect that some people experience is the lightening or disappearance of their period altogether.

Things to remember:

- When the patch is used consistently and correctly, it can be 99% effective at preventing pregnancy. However, using the patch flawlessly isn't always what happens. Because people can make mistakes when using the patch, the typical effectiveness is 91%.

- Only female-bodied people can use the patch

- The patch does not prevent the transmission of STIs

- You have to have a prescription for the patch

- The patch ranges in cost from $0-$100

The Ring

"The ring" (also known by its manufacturer's name, NuvaRing) is a hormonal contraception method that is inserted into the vagina. It is made of bendable plastic and the user inserts it into the vagina and leaves it alone for a month. Like the other hormonal contraception we have already

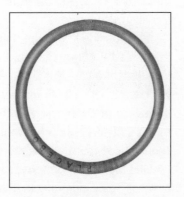

The ring is extremely flexible in order to be easily inserted into the vagina.

gone over, it requires a prescription from a health care provider and works in the same way: by preventing ovulation (the release of an egg) and thickening the cervical mucus (preventing sperm from entering the uterus). The ring is most effective when it's used consistently and correctly. Meaning, it's inserted as close to the cervix as possible and is changed at the same time monthly. Unlike some of the other forms of contraception, this method requires the user to be comfortable with their body since they will need to insert their fingers into the vagina.

Because the ring doesn't need to be thought about daily or even weekly, it's suggested that the user mark their calendar or set up a reminder in their phone so that they remember to change their ring on time. This can look different for different people. The user has the option of leaving the ring in for four weeks, removing the ring and immediately inserting another ring to skip a period, or the user can leave the ring out a week which will allow for the user to have their monthly period, and after leaving the ring out of the body for a week, inserting a new ring. A lot of users really like this feature.

If you decide to use the ring, you can start it at any point. If you start it during the first five days of your period, it's effective right away. But if you start it at any other point, you will need to use a back-up method, like a condom. Typically, a medical provider will give the user at least three rings to have on hand (if not a full year's worth). Storage for the ring should be at room temperature.

Like the other hormonal contraception methods, the ring also has some side effects that typically go away after using it for two to three months. Side effects are usually headaches, feeling sick to the stomach, and irregular periods and/

or spotting. Many users report that after six months of use, their periods become really light or go away completely when the ring is used for four weeks straight (without the one week off). [35]

A common question asked about the ring is, "Can the ring fall out?" Not likely. Remember when we talked about anatomy, we said that the vagina is a muscle? Those muscles will work to keep the ring in place. Sometimes people develop more discharge with the ring. This is normal and will act as a natural lubrication, which can increase the chance that the ring will fall out. But, don't stress if it does come out. The user will still be protected from pregnancy as long as it has been out of the body for less than two days (and it's not a ring-free week). If the ring falls out of the body, wash it off with cool water (not warm or hot) and put it back in. Easy-peasy. You'll definitely want to use a back-up method just to be sure for the next seven days though.

Another concern folks have about the ring is if they forget to change it—what happens? Nothing bad! You will just want to change it as soon as you remember, use a back-up method, and change your schedule to reflect the new insertion date (i.e. change the ring after this three weeks from the date of insertion).

When you insert a new ring, hold on to the packaging. This is where you are going to want to dispose of the old ring. Just take the ring out of the body, put it in the package, seal it up, and you're good to go. Never put a ring in the toilet, as this will clog it. Always throw it in the trash.

---

35 "How Do I Start Using NuvaRing?" Planned Parenthood. Accessed July 19, 2018. https://www.plannedparenthood.org/learn/birth-control/birth-control-vaginal-ring-nuvaring/how-do-i-start-using-nuvaring

Things to remember:

- When the ring is used consistently and correctly, it can be 99% effective at preventing pregnancy. However, using the ring flawlessly isn't always what happens. Because people can make mistakes when using the ring, the typical effectiveness is 91%.

- Only female-bodied people can use the ring

- The ring does not prevent the transmission of STIs

- You have to have a prescription for the ring

- The ring ranges in cost from $0-$200

The Diaphragm

A flexible, latex-looking cup, the diaphragm has been around for a long time. It's something that you need to see a health care provider for, so they can measure your cervix to ensure that the diaphragm fits well. Fitting correctly is part of correct and consistent use to ensure that it is effective. It also needs to be used with spermicide (we'll go into what this is in a few).

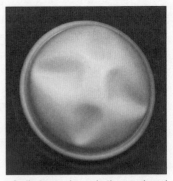

A diaphragm is a plastic cup-shaped device that is flexible so that it can be easily inserted into the vagina. The rim of a diaphragm should be covered with spermicide to make it most effective at preventing pregnancy.

Like the ring, the user needs to feel comfortable inserting their fingers into their vagina so that they can ensure proper placement. To insert it, you bend it like the ring and place it up against the cervix. But before you insert it, you will line the rim with spermicide.

Unlike the ring, the diaphragm is not a hormonal form of contraception. It's what is called a "barrier method." That means that instead of preventing ovulation, it acts as a wall blocking the entry of sperm into the uterus. Because there are no hormones, side effects are rare. If you have a latex allergy, you won't be able to use a diaphragm, and some people become irritated by the chemicals in the spermicide (usually this presents as increased discharge and/or itchiness and may result in a yeast infection).

What's a yeast infection? A yeast infection is a very common infection that most female-bodied people get at some point in their life according to the U.S. Department of Health and Human Services. [36] It's basically caused by an imbalance of bacteria in the vagina that leads to burning, itching and increased discharge that can also be a different color and smell than usual. Yeast infections are pretty easy to get rid of, but it's still important to see a medical professional if you see these types of symptoms so that they can accurately diagnose what you have (making sure it isn't something else) and give you the proper medication, whether that's a prescription or over the counter medicine.

Because a diaphragm needs to fit perfectly to be the most effective, it isn't always a good option for teenagers. Remember, as a teenager, your body is still growing and developing. And since your cervix is inside your body, it isn't easy to tell if it's changing. Therefore, you can't be sure that the diaphragm

---

36 "Vaginal yeast infections." Womenshealth.gov. April 18, 2017. Accessed January 17, 2018. http://www.womenshealth.gov/a-z-topics/vaginal-yeast-infections.

is fitting correctly unless you're regularly seeing a health care provider. And let's be honest, who wants to head to the clinic every month or so for a measurement of their cervix?

A diaphragm can be inserted up to two hours before you have sex. It can stay in if you're going to have sex again soon after, but you would need to reapply the spermicide and wait until the spermicide is effective (it will say on the directions of the spermicide). After you have had sex, you will want to leave it in your body for at least six hours, but no more than 24 hours.

If you decide to use a diaphragm, you will only have one because after each use you will remove it, wash it, and then store it in the case it comes in. You will want to store it at room temperature and make sure the soap you use is gentle. Always let your diaphragm air dry and regularly check it for holes or tears. You can use water to see if there is a leak you can't see. If there is, don't use it (use something else), and you will need to get another one from your medical provider.

Things to remember:

- When a diaphragm is used consistently and correctly, it can be 94% effective at preventing pregnancy. However, using a diaphragm flawlessly isn't always what happens. Because people can make mistakes, the typical effectiveness is 88%.

- Only female-bodied people can use the diaphragm

- The diaphragm does not prevent the transmission of STIs

- You need to see a health care provider to get a diaphragm

- Diaphragms range in cost from $0-$75

The Male Condom

The what? Yeah, that's right. What is commonly called a "condom" I am actually calling a "male condom." That is because there is also a thing out there called "the female condom." I'm going to go into what this is next. For now, let's focus on the male condom. One of the oldest known forms of contraception, the male condom has been around for a *long* time. That's because it's pretty darn effective at keeping people from becoming pregnant. You know what else? It's also super great at preventing STI transmission.

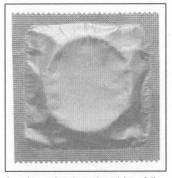

A male condom is packaged in a foil or plastic wrapping.

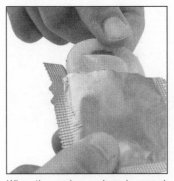

When the condom package is opened, it needs to be carefully pulled out of the package. The condom itself is most commonly made out of a really flexible plastic called latex.

The male condom is meant to be worn by a male-bodied person and comes in different colors, sizes, flavors, textures and materials. They can be purchased at grocery stores, online, at convenience stores, and in public bathroom dispensers, or found in health care facilities (among other places). Male condoms can be used to protect individuals during vaginal, anal, and oral sex. (Obviously, it's only preventing pregnancy during vaginal sex. If you need a refresher on this, go to chapter

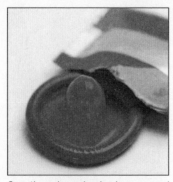

Once the male condom has been removed from the package, you can see there is a little tip on the end that sort-of looks like a hat. The condom is designed in this way so that the user can tell which way it should be put on the penis or sex toy, and so it can be rolled down smoothly. That little tip is designed to catch the ejaculation from the penis.

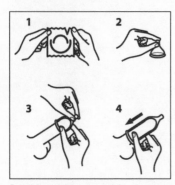

Practicing putting on a condom is a great way to make sure that it's going to be effective at protecting you and your partner. You don't need a penis to practice! Try practicing on a cucumber or banana.

14.) In fact, that is why there are so many different kinds of condoms out there.

Most condoms are made out of a thin rubber called latex. The male condom is designed to be put on the penis when it's erect and kept on the penis until after ejaculation. The male condom is effective because it acts as a barrier between the partners: it keeps the penis and the penis's fluids separate from the vagina and vaginal fluids (or anus or mouth).

Because there are so many different kinds of male condoms out there, choosing the right one for you can be a little intimidating. First, start with what kind of sex you're going to be having. If you're having oral sex, you might want to choose a male condom that is flavored. These are specially designed just for oral sex and are covered with a sugary substance that gives them their flavor. You wouldn't want to use a flavored condom for vaginal or anal sex. The sugary substance that gives it its flavor can cause an irritation or infection in the anus or vagina.

If you're engaging in anal or vaginal sex, you are going to look at non-flavored condoms. The color or texture of a condom you choose is based purely on what you like and what feels good to you and your partner. As for size, let's get real. The typical condom fits everyone. Sure, for some people it might feel a little snug (for which there are bigger sizes available), but a typical condom can, and will, fit any penis. How do I know? Well, try this out for yourself. Get a condom and gently roll it over your hand. Seriously. Do it. I'll wait.

See? It stretches. While it might be nice to think your's or your partner's penis needs a bigger-sized male condom, chances are, you don't. In fact, wearing a larger-sized condom can actually put you at risk for the condom coming out during sexual activity. And if that happens? You aren't going to be protected.

As for materials, this is something that you want to pay attention to. As I said, the most common material out there is latex. If you or your partner have a latex allergy, though, definitely *don't* use a latex condom. You will want to choose a condom made from plastic (either polyurethane, nitrile, or polyisoprene) or lambskin. The plastic condoms aren't as stretchy as a latex or lambskin condom, and lambskin condoms aren't as effective in preventing STI transmission. But they all are equal in preventing pregnancy when used consistently and correctly.

As with other forms of contraception, if you want them to be most effective, you want to follow the directions carefully. For male condoms, you might even want to practice putting it on (either on a penis or something penis-like, like a banana) so that you're comfortable using a condom before you get into a sexual situation. Even though the male condom is for a male-bodied person to wear, it's also good for female-bodied people to know how to use them. Even if you don't think you'll be engaging in sex with a male-bodied person, you might use sex toys that are penis shaped and can practice safer sex by covering the toys with a male condom (especially if you're sharing sex toys with a partner). Or you might have friends who have sex with male-bodied people and you can help them be safe as well!

In order for condoms to be the most effective at preventing pregnancy and STI transmission, the condom needs to go on the penis (or toy) *before* it comes into contact with the partner's vagina, mouth, or anus and after the penis becomes erect. If you're using a condom on a penis, by waiting until the penis is erect, you can ensure you're putting it on correctly (plus it will be easier). You want to put the condom on the penis before it contacts a partner's vagina, mouth, or anus because it can protect you and your partner from STIs that are transmitted from skin to skin contact, and it also ensures your partner doesn't come into contact with pre-ejaculate or "pre-cum." If you need a refresher on that, go to page 56.

Here are the steps that will help ensure you're using male condoms correctly and consistently:

Before you have sexual contact (this could be even before you go out for the night) check the expiration date. Just like milk, condoms have expiration dates. You wouldn't drink milk that is expired so don't use a condom that has expired. The expiration date will be printed on the individual package as well as the box. If it isn't expired, you can use it!

Another cool thing about condoms? They can be used with another form of contraception like the pill or IUD to increase pregnancy protection! "Dual method use offers protection against both pregnancy and STIs. In 2006–2010, one in five sexually active females aged fifteen to nineteen and one-third of sexually active males in this age-group said that they used both a condom and a hormonal method the last time they had sex."[37]

Now it's time to open the condom package. While you might think it will look sexy to open a condom package with your teeth—don't. In fact, don't use anything sharp to open a condom package (like scissors). If you use something sharp like scissors or your teeth, you run the risk of cutting or tearing the actual condom and not just the package, which will make the condom unusable. Use the pads of your fingers to gently tear open the package. Once you've opened the package, pull the condom out of the package and look at it. See any tears or holes? If yes, toss it. If no, let's move on to the next step.

This is where you're going to put the condom on the penis (or sex toy). Before setting the condom on the penis, check which way the condom is going to roll. The rim of the condom should be on the outside and it should look like a little hat. Go ahead and unroll it a little. Is it easy to unroll? If yes, proceed to the next step. If not, flip it inside out and then proceed to the next step. If you forgot to check the way it rolls and you put it on the tip of the penis inside out, toss

37   Martinez G et al., Teenagers in the United States: sexual activity, contraceptive use, and childbearing, 2006–2010 National Survey of Family Growth, Vital and Health Statistics, 2011, Series 23, No. 31.

it. By placing it on the tip of the penis, any pre-ejaculate or STI present may have gotten on the tip of the condom. The tip that, once you flip it inside out, would go into your partner. That defeats the purpose and you'll need to start over with a new, fresh condom. (See, this is why it's good to practice.)

Okay. You know which way the condom is supposed to roll, so let's put it on the penis. Gently squeeze the tip of the condom. You want to do this to ensure that there is room at the tip of the condom in what is called the "reservoir" to contain the ejaculate or semen. If the male using the condom is uncircumcised, they (or their partner) will want to pull the foreskin of the penis back a little before placing the condom on the tip of the penis. Now go ahead and unroll the condom down the shaft of the penis. You will want to make sure the condom is completely unrolled. If the condom feels tight while it's being rolled down, it's okay to add a couple drops of lubrication as long as it is water-based lubricant. (Using anything but water-based lubrication can break down the material of the condom and make it ineffective.) Once the condom is on, you can also add some lubrication to the outside of the condom. (This is especially important for anal sex—refer to page 118 for more on lubrication.)

Have sex!

After the male-bodied person ejaculates, they will want to hold on to the base of the condom as they pull out of their partner. If you're using a condom on a sex toy, you will want to hold onto the base of the condom on the sex toy, even though there isn't semen present. Holding on to the base of the condom as the penis or sex toy is pulled out ensures that the condom comes out with the penis or sex toy and doesn't stay in your partner.

To remove the condom from the penis, the male-bodied person will want to turn away from their partner so that nothing accidently spills out onto their partner. Then they will want to wrap the condom up and throw it away. Never throw a condom down a toilet because this will clog your toilet.

Male condoms are a one-time use method of contraception and STI prevention. If you're going to be having different kinds of sex, use a different condom for each type. For example, if you're switching between vaginal and anal sex, use a different condom for each (this is true whether it's a penis or a sex toy) to ensure that the condom is clean and to avoid infections. Use it once and then toss it. Also, as we've mentioned, male condoms are a great back-up method for hormonal contraception. But *never* use two condoms together. This actually weakens the effectiveness because they will be more susceptible to breaks or tears.

Things to remember:

> **FUN FACT:** Condoms don't have any side effects!

- When condoms are used consistently and correctly, they can be 98% effective at preventing pregnancy. However, using condoms flawlessly isn't always what happens. Because people can make mistakes when using condoms, the typical effectiveness is 82%.

- The condom can be used on a penis or sex toy (and is the only form of contraception specifically designed for the male body)

- The condom does prevent the transmission of STIs
- You can get condoms almost anywhere
- Condoms range in cost from $0-$2

The Female Condom

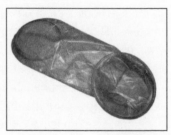

Yes. You read that correctly. There is such a thing as a female condom. They are pretty hard to find, but they are out there, and they are almost as effective as the male condom in preventing pregnancy and STI transmission. Instead of being

The female condom is much larger and less stretchy than a male condom.

worn by a person with a penis (or put on a sex toy), this one is used inside the body. So, it's designed to go inside the vagina or anus. These types of condoms are also called "internal condoms" (and the male condom can be called the "external condom"). As of publication, there is only one brand of female condom, the FC2 Female Condom. Unlike the male condom, there is just the one brand and it's only one material—plastic (nitrile). Just like the male condom, the female condom acts as a barrier and prevents the sperm from meeting the egg so there isn't a pregnancy. It also covers skin and prevents skin-to-skin contact, so it can be a great option in preventing STI transmission.

If you're interested in using a female condom, you don't need a prescription, but they can be a little tricky to find. You can definitely get them online and at various health care providers. As more people use them, they can be found at some pharmacies or grocery stores. Some people prefer the female condom over the male condom because, if they are engaging in heterosexual sex, they don't have to rely on their partner to remember the condom—they take the power back! And many folks say that penis-to-vagina sex is more comfortable when using the female condom because it's looser than a male condom. Another cool thing about the female condom is that it can be put in the vagina before you and your partner start messing around. So, there isn't any need to stop when things are getting hot. Also, the female condom doesn't have any side effects, so, you know, that's cool, too.

When using a female condom, the instructions are really similar to using a male condom. (I'm going to explain how you use a female condom as if it's being inserted into the vagina.)

First, you're going to want to check the expiration date on the condom. Each condom has the expiration date printed on the package and the box.

You will then want to open the package (remember, no fancy stuff here, just use the pads of your fingers).

The female condom comes pre-lubricated so there isn't really a need to add more lubrication. But if you want to you can.

Then, you (or your partner) are going to bend the plastic loop inside the female condom so it fits inside the vagina. You (or your partner) will want to push it up as far as it can go, ideally so that the plastic ring is resting against the cervix. If you (or your partner) can't get it up that far with your fingers, don't stress! When the penis goes into the female condom, it will push it into the vagina farther. Remember, it can't "get lost up there" because your cervix will prevent anything from going into your uterus. In order to get it up as far as it can go with your fingers, think about what it's like to put in a tampon or the menstrual cup. You want to get in a position with your legs spread as you lie down or with one foot elevated as you stand.

Make sure the ring doesn't twist as you insert it!

The whole condom isn't going to go inside the vagina. You will want to leave the end ring out of the vagina (about an inch). It's this extra plastic on the female condom that makes it a favorite among some folks – that extra plastic gives a little extra coverage for the vulva when it comes to skin-to-skin contact.

Because the female condom fits a little looser than the male condom, the users should make sure that the penis goes inside the female condom and doesn't go on the side of the female condom. Because, well, this is going to produce more of a risk for pregnancy and STI transmission. Even if it's an "oops," and you fix the position, the penis has entered the vagina without protection and, if there is pre-ejaculate (or pre-cum) there is a risk for pregnancy. And obviously, the skin-to-skin contact and/or pre-ejaculate increases a risk for STI transmission.

Once the penis is in the female condom, go ahead and do your thing (just check to make sure the penis stays inside the female condom during the entire sex act),

Once you're finished, pull the penis out of the female condom, twist the outside ring (so nothing comes out) and pull. Wrap the used female condom in toilet paper or it's plastic package and throw it away.

If you're going to use the female condom for anal sex, the

inner ring should be removed before you use it and it should be inserted into the anus with your finger (making sure the external ring stays outside the body).

Things to remember:

- When female condoms are used consistently and correctly, they can be 95% effective at preventing pregnancy. However, using female condoms flaw-lessly isn't always what happens. Because people can make mistakes, the typical effectiveness is 79%.

- The female condom can be used in the vagina or anus

- The female condom does prevent the transmission of STIs

- Condoms cost about $0-$2

A female condom has a one-time use and should not be used with a male condom. Using two condoms together makes them less effective!

Withdrawal

The withdrawal method refers to removing the penis from the vagina before ejaculation and is also called "the pull-out method." The withdrawal method does not protect against the transmission of STIs because there is no barrier between the penis and vagina. The risk for pregnancy in this method is higher for a couple of reasons. First, a male-bodied person cannot feel pre-cum or pre-ejaculate leaving the penis. This pre-cum can contain sperm. Second, not all male-bodied people know exactly when they are going to ejaculate. (This is especially true for male-bodied people who aren't as familiar with their bodies.) So, a male-bodied person may try to withdraw the penis from the vagina but not fully remove the penis before ejaculating. Remember, even if semen gets on the edge of the vaginal opening or on the vulva, there is still a risk for pregnancy. There are no side effects of the withdrawal method.

Things to remember:

- Because people don't always use the withdrawal method flawlessly, the typical effectiveness is 78% for withdrawal (meaning fully withdrawn prior to ejaculation)
- Withdrawal can be used for anal, oral, and vaginal sex
- Withdrawal does not prevent the transmission of STIs
- Withdrawal is free

Sponge

The sponge is made out of soft plastic that looks and feels a lot like a sponge (thus the name). The name brand for the sponge is the "Today Sponge." The sponge can be purchased online and it can be found at some pharmacies and grocery stores. You don't need a prescription to use it.

Each sponge is designed to be inserted only once, but can be inside the body before having sex, so there is no need to interrupt what's going on with your partner to ensure you're protected. Check the instructions to see how many hours in advance of sex the sponge can be inserted. Also, once the sponge is in the body, you can have sex more than once and count on it being just as effective as the first time you had sex. Here's the kicker, though—it needs to stay in the body for at least six hours after the last instance of sex. If it's removed before the six hours are up, it will not be as effective. Also, once it's used and taken out, you have to use a new one as each sponge is only good for 24 hours once it has been "activated" (or gotten wet and inserted into the vagina).

The sponge works by being put into the vagina as far as it goes, so the user is going to need to be comfortable with their body. It's made to cover up the cervix and contains spermicide. It acts as a partial barrier to the uterus, preventing sperm from entering the body, and the spermicide slows down or kills the sperm. The sponge does not protect from the transmission of STIs, but is effective against pregnancy as soon as it's inserted into the body. You can definitely use the sponge with a condom though for extra pregnancy protection and to prevent the transmission of STIs.

If you want to use the sponge, you need to use it correctly for it to be the most effective at preventing pregnancy. Because you're going to be inserting the sponge into your body, make sure your hands are clean and then wet the sponge. Give it a couple squeezes so that the spermicide is activated (bubbles and foam will start to come out). You will then fold the sponge and, with the little stringy thing facing out, insert the sponge into the vagina. Inserting the sponge into the vagina is a lot like putting in a tampon, so positioning your body in a similar way (laying down or squatting or elevating one of your legs) will help you be more comfortable as you insert it. As you insert it, push it up as far as it can go with your fingers, and it will unfold as you get it into place, with your vaginal muscles holding it in place. Just make sure your cervix is covered by feeling the edges of the sponge.

When you're done having sex and six hours have passed, you're ready to remove the sponge. Again, making sure your hands are clean, put your finger inside your vagina and pull the sponge out using that little string that is attached to the sponge. If the string has been pushed up against the body or you can't find it, don't panic. Using your finger, just grab the edge of the sponge and gently pull it down. Once it's out of the body, make sure you wrap it up in some toilet paper and throw it in the trash—never flush it down the toilet because it will cause your toilet to back up.

Some people do experience side effects from the sponge. Because the chemical spermicide is in the sponge, some people are allergic to it or find the chemicals irritating. Also, it's not recommended to use the sponge if you're having your period because it can increase your risk of toxic shock syndrome.

What's Toxic Shock Syndrome? TSS, or Toxic Shock Syndrome, is something that can happen to female-bodied people who leave something (like the sponge or a tampon) inside the vagina for too long. It's a rare problem, especially if the user adheres to the directions of tampon and sponge use. It's basically a dangerous overgrowth of bacteria in the vagina. Symptoms include vomiting, diarrhea, a sunburn-like rash and a high fever. If you're experiencing symptoms like this and have used a tampon or the sponge, see a medical provider immediately. TSS is really dangerous.

Things to remember:

- Because people don't always use the sponge flawlessly, the typical effectiveness is 76-88%

- No prescription is needed for the sponge

- The sponge does not prevent the transmission of STIs

- The sponge costs up to $15 for a pack of 3

Fertility Awareness Method

The Fertility Awareness Method, or FAM, is a way to prevent pregnancy that relies on the tracking of your menstrual cycle. It's also called "natural family planning," "the rhythm method," and "the calendar method." There are a couple of different ways to do this, but they all require understanding when you're most fertile (ovulating) and strictly adhering to abstinence during that time period. There are three ways to try to figure out when you're most fertile. You can take your basal temperature (this is your resting temperature, taken first thing in the morning before you wake up), you can check your daily discharge or cervical mucus, and/or you can chart your menstrual cycle with an app or calendar. To make FAM most effective, it's suggested you use all three methods.

Calendar method

It may look easy, but there is a lot of tracking that needs to be done in order to be as accurate as possible in understanding your menstrual cycle.

While these methods are free or relatively inexpensive, they are extremely difficult for teens to use. The biggest challenge is that a teen's menstrual cycle may not be very regular due to the changes a teen experiences with their hormones. Most female-bodied teens have irregular periods, meaning that the flow can change from month to month, as can the number of days between periods. If you want to use FAM, you're going to want to speak with a medical provider who can instruct you on the necessary steps. Also, in order to really know your cycle, it's recommended that you track your menstrual cycle for at least six months before relying on it as a form of contraception to ensure you know the pattern of your body.

Things to remember:

- Because people don't always use FAM flawlessly, the typical effectiveness is 76%

- FAM does not prevent the transmission of STIs

- FAM can cost up to $20 for supplies

Spermicide

Spermicide is a chemical that is put into the vagina prior to sex. There are lots of different kinds of spermicide out there. They come in gels, foams, suppositories, even film. But they all work in the same way to prevent pregnancy—by disabling the ability for the sperm to swim and blocking the cervical opening. Spermicide can be used on its own but it doesn't prevent the transmission of STIs. Spermicide can also be used with a condom for extra pregnancy and STI protection or with another form of contraception to increase its effectiveness. Because there are several different kinds and brands of spermicide out there, it's critically important that you read the instructions for how to use it. Each one will be a little different, and the time you need to wait to ensure they are as effective as possible also varies depending on the kind you're using. One thing is the same: you want to get the spermicide as close to the cervix as possible to make it as effective as possible.

Spermicide is pretty easy to find. You can get it at the grocery store or pharmacy and you don't need a prescription. Spermicide also has very few side effects (unless you're allergic to the chemicals in the spermicide). Some people report that their vagina or penis becomes irritated from the chemicals, but this irritation typically goes away on its own. It's important to note that if you or your partner are irritated by the chemicals in spermicide, you can actually be more at risk for contracting an STI if you're exposed to an STI. That's because the irritation actually makes it easier for the STI germs to enter the body (because it's like an open wound). The biggest complaint users of spermicide have is that it can be messy. Also, if a person tries to have oral sex with the vagina after spermicide is used, the spermicide can get in their mouth—

which doesn't taste good, and depending on whether it is swallowed (and how much), it can even make you feel sick.

Things to remember:

- Because people don't always use spermicide flawlessly, the typical effectiveness is 72%
- Spermicide does not prevent the transmission of STIs
- Spermicide can cost up to $8

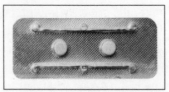

No matter how careful you are, there can still be something that goes wrong. Emergency Contraception is a great option to try and prevent a pregnancy after sex.

Whoops!
Sometimes, no matter how careful you are, a mistake happens—the condom breaks, or after having sex you realize you missed a pill. Maybe you weren't planning on having sex and weren't prepared, but decided to have sex anyway. (Or maybe you were coerced or forced to have sex against your will, which is *not* okay. Please go to chapter 18 for more information and resources.) There is another option that works to prevent pregnancy after unprotected sex. It's called emergency contraception. "A survey conducted from 2011 to 2013 showed that, among females ages fifteen to nineteen who have had sexual intercourse, twenty-two percent said they had used emergency contraception at least once in their lives."[38] Emergency

38 Rettner, Rachael. "More Teens Use 'Morning-After Pill,' Study Finds." LiveScience. July 22, 2015. Accessed July 17, 2018. https://www.livescience.com/51622-teens-emergency-contraception-increase.html.

contraception, or EC, or Plan B, is *not* abortion. In fact, if you're already pregnant, taking EC will not affect your pregnancy.

There are two forms of EC: first, you can see a health care provider and have an IUD inserted within 120 hours—that's five days—after unprotected sex. This is the most effective type of EC. And the sooner you have the IUD inserted, the more effective it will be. This type of EC works in the same way to prevent pregnancy as any IUD (check out page 170).

The second type of EC is a medication that comes in a pill form. If you're interested in the pill form of EC (also called the morning-after pill), you need to know that there are two kinds available: one made out of ulipristal acetate and one made out of levonorgestrel. The only pill made out of ulipristal acete is called Ella, and you need to have a prescription for it. You can order it online, or you can get it at a pharmacy or health clinic like Planned Parenthood. This is the most effective form of medication EC and can be taken within 120 hours (five days) of unprotected sex.

The other form of medication EC with levonorgestrel is easier to get. You don't need a prescription, and there are several different brand names, including Plan B One-Step and AfterPill. Again, this medication must be taken within five days of unprotected sex (or 120 hours) but it's most effective when taken within 72 hours (or three days) after unprotected sex. You'll find this version of EC at a drug store or health care clinic. The bottom line with EC is the sooner you take it (or have it inserted if you're going the IUD route), the more effective it is at preventing pregnancy. Both of these pills work similarly to hormonal contraception by thickening the cervical mucus and preventing ovulation (the release of an egg). If the sperm has already met the egg, these medications will not end a pregnancy.

If you decide to use medication EC, side effects are rare. Some female-bodied people report feeling nauseous or dizzy, or even having a headache. These symptoms are the result of a large amount of hormones entering your body at one time, and they are temporary. Also, because taking medication EC will trigger your body to have a period when it wasn't planning on it, you might notice that your period flow is a little different than usual or that you have more intense cramps. Your period should go back to normal following the EC-stimulated cycle, but your menstrual cycle will now follow the induced period's schedule. In other words, when you are mapping out your menstrual cycle, you will now move forward using the end date of the EC-induced period.

EC is called emergency contraception because it's designed to be used in the case of an emergency. While taking EC whenever you need it isn't bad for your body, it isn't something you should rely on for primary prevention of pregnancy for a couple of reasons: it's expensive (an IUD can cost anywhere from $0-$1,000 and the pills can range in cost from $20-50 per dose), there are side effects (like feeling sick to your stomach and/or headaches if you take a pill form of EC) and it doesn't work as well as other contraception methods out there (like the IUD, pill, shot, etc.). So, definitely use EC if you need to, but think about it as, well, something to use in an emergency.

FUN FACT: Did you know that an IUD can also be used as emergency contraception? It's a good option for female-bodied people who have a sensitivity to hormones. If an IUD is inserted after unprotected sex, it can prevent a pregnancy from happening if it is inserted within five days after unprotected sex.

What is a dental dam? A dental dam is a rectangular piece of latex that can cover the vaginal or anal opening. It's used for oral sex and protects from STIs. A dental dam does not protect against pregnancy. Dental dams aren't the easiest to find. Sex stores have them and they can also be found online. If you don't have access to a dental dam, you can cut up a flavored condom or even use saran wrap or a plastic bag. Just make sure that you use each piece of plastic only one time and that the part of the material that touched the genitals doesn't end up in your mouth.

If you want to try and figure out what the best method is for you before you go in to see a medical professional, there's an app for that. Planned Parenthood has developed an app called "Spot On." The app is designed to help the user determine what contraception is best for them, track their menstrual cycle, and remember to take or use their contraception. Technology is awesome!

CONVERSATION STARTERS . . .

• • • • • • • • • •

The conversation starters are designed to be prompts for having conversations. Feel free to use them in the way that feels right to you.

Questions for Teens to Ask Their Parents

- Have you ever used contraception? What kinds? What was your experience?

- Do we have insurance that will cover contraception? Do we have a co-pay?

- Have you ever had a "whoops"? What happened? What did you do? Why did you make that decision?

Questions for Parents to Ask Their Teens

- Do you think you're ready to get on or purchase contraception? Would you like to talk to a medical provider about starting contraception? (Remember, being on contraception does NOT mean a person is sexually active.)

- Do you need help determining what contraception is going to be best for you?

15

WHAT IF THERE'S A PREGNANCY?

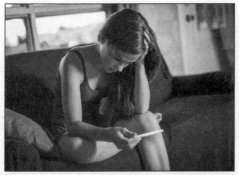

Whether your contraceptive method failed, you forgot to use it, or you were forced to have sex, unplanned pregnancies happen. Becoming pregnant has a major impact on your life. You need to know what your options are and how you feel about them. And remember, until it happens to you, you can never know what you might do. Whatever you do, don't make a decision on your own. Talk to your partner and your parents or another trusted adult. Get the facts and make a decision based on what is best for you. It's your body.

No matter how well you plan and protect yourself, you or your partner might become pregnant if you are sexually active. Seventy-five percent of teen pregnancies are unintended[39] meaning the people involved were actively trying

39 Finer LB and Zolna MR, Declines in unintended pregnancy in the United States, 2008–2011, New England Journal of Medicine, 2016, 374(9):843–852.

to *not* become pregnant. In 2011, about 553,000 U.S. women aged fifteen to nineteen became pregnant with 70% of those teen pregnancies occurring among eighteen to nineteen-year-olds. [40] Remember, the only way to make sure you and your partner do not get pregnant is to not have sex (practicing abstinence). But, if you do find that you're pregnant, you've got some options. You can choose to parent. You can choose adoption. Or you can choose abortion. If you are the person who is pregnant, only you can decide which is the best option for you. Should you become pregnant, talk with your partner, family, and other mentors. They can help you with your decision. For some people, the decision is easy. For others, not so much. Before you engage in sex, you definitely want to consider what you might do if you or your partner became pregnant. Even if you think you're being safe or engaging in sex that can't result in a pregnancy, or if you identify as homosexual, it's important to consider all the risks.

Did you know that gay and bisexual youth experience pregnancy at a higher rate than heterosexual teens? [41] Many studies suggest that youth who are LGBTQ+ are more likely to start having sex before their peers. They also tend to have more partners and use alcohol and drugs when having sex, but are less likely to use protection like condoms. But why? It has nothing to do with the way they identify and everything to do with how society marginalizes the LGBTQ+ population. Without a supportive environment, LGBTQ+ youth are at greater risk for experiencing harmful behaviors like bullying

40 Kost K and Maddow-Zimet I, U.S. Teenage Pregnancies, Births and Abortions, 2011: National Trends by Age, Race and Ethnicity, New York: Guttmacher Institute, 2016
41 "Pregnancies more common among lesbian, gay, bisexual youths." Reuters. May 14, 2015. Accessed January 17, 2018. http://www.reuters.com/article/us-pregnancy-teen-lgbt/pregnancies-more-common-among-lesbian-gay-bisexual-youths-idUSKBN0NZ2AT20150514.

and partner violence. As a result, someone who is LGBTQ+ may then engage in more risky sexual behaviors, like not using contraception or STI protection. [42]

There are so many things that go into a person's decision about how they want to handle a pregnancy. Unless you have been in the same situation as the person who is pregnant, you can't know what their life circumstances are and what their decision-making process is. Ultimately, it's their body and they get to make the decisions. [43]

PARENTING

If you decide to parent the child, you're deciding to carry the pregnancy until birth and then be a parent to the child for the child's entire life. You will need to think about how being pregnant and having a child will impact your life. Have you ever thought about whether you want to be a parent? How will it change your goals? Do you have a partner who is committed to helping raise the child? Where will you live? How will you pay for food, clothes, medicine, etc.? Do you have family and friends who are supportive?

If, after considering the above questions, you decide you want to parent, and you're carrying the fetus (a developing baby), you are going to want to seek medical care right away. When you're pregnant, it's important that you and the fetus receive proper medical care. This includes making

42 Charlton, B. M., H. L. Corliss, S. A. Missmer, M. Rosario, D. Spiegelman, and S. B. Austin. "Sexual orientation differences in teen pregnancy and hormonal contraceptive use: an examination across 2 generations." American journal of obstetrics and gynecology. September 2013. Accessed January 17, 2018. http://www.ncbi.nlm.nih.gov/pubmed/23796650

43 Kost K and Maddow-Zimet I, U.S. Teenage Pregnancies, Births and Abortions, 2011: National Trends by Age, Race and Ethnicity, New York: Guttmacher Institute, 2016.

sure you cease drinking alcohol, smoking, and taking drugs. It also means getting the right amount of exercise, proper nutrition, and staying hydrated. Prenatal vitamins are also recommended.

ADOPTION

Adoption is an option if you become pregnant and don't want to parent. Adoption means that you will deliver the baby and the adoptive parents will raise the child. There are many forms of adoptions. With some adoptions, you choose the parents/family for the child and are able to be in some kind of contact with the family and/or child throughout their life. This contact can vary and often the terms of the adoptive relationship can be negotiated to meet both parties' needs. With other adoptions, the child has no contact with the birth parent. Again, if this is the route you decide to go down, you need to think about what is right for you and your life. Only you can decide what relationship you are comfortable with.

ABORTION

Abortion is the ending of a pregnancy or termination of a pregnancy. Abortion has been legal in the United States since 1973 as a result of a Supreme Court case called Roe vs. Wade. This decision by the Supreme Court stated that a female-bodied person who is pregnant has the right to decide whether they want to be pregnant or legally terminate the pregnancy. Up until this time, abortions were still happening, but they were happening illegally and often with dire consequences for the woman, such as death or infertility.

When abortion became legal, it meant that doctors and nurse practitioners could offer abortion safely. While laws differ from state to state on how far along a person can be when they get an abortion or what that person must do before getting an abortion, it's still safe and legal in the United States. In 2011, over 142,600 abortions were had by women aged fifteen to nineteen. That's approximately five percent of all abortions that year.[44] Whether or not a person chooses abortion, it is an extremely personal choice, and everyone's reasons are different. The reasons teens most frequently give for having an abortion are concerns about how having a baby would change their lives, inability to afford a baby, and not wanting to be a single mother.[45] Deciding to have an abortion is an easy choice for some people, while others might struggle. Sometimes female-bodied people struggle because they want children, but not right now. They may feel that it is against their religion, or they may take into account that they have a strong support system that can help raise the child. There are many factors that go into an individual's choice, and every person's situation is different. Only those involved know what is best for them.[46]

Finding an abortion provider can be challenging depending on where you live. And even if abortion is available, you may need your parents to be involved. As of August 2016, laws in thirty-seven states required that a minor seeking an abortion involve one or both parents in the decision.[47]

44 Kost K and Maddow-Zimet I, U.S. Teenage Pregnancies, Births and Abortions, 2011: National Trends by Age, Race and Ethnicity, New York: Guttmacher Institute, 2016.
45 Finer LB et al., Reasons U.S. women have abortions: quantitative and qualitative perspectives, Perspectives on Sexual and Reproductive Health, 2005, 37(3):110–118.
46 Kost K and Maddow-Zimet I, U.S. Teenage Pregnancies, Births and Abortions, 2011: National Trends by Age, Race and Ethnicity, New York: Guttmacher Institute, 2016.
47 "Parental Involvement in Minors' Abortions." Guttmacher Institute. January 02, 2018. Accessed January 17, 2018. https://www.guttmacher.org/state-policy/explore/parental-involvement-minors-abortions.

Additionally, there are many providers who will not complete an abortion if you're more than 12 weeks pregnant. If you decide you want an abortion, it is best to get it as soon as you can upon finding out you're pregnant. There are two types of abortions available in the United States: surgical (or in-clinic) abortions and medication abortions.

IN-CLINIC ABORTION

An in-clinic abortion ends a pregnancy by physically removing the fetus from the uterus. This can be done through a procedure called vacuum aspiration or suction. This type of procedure can be done on a female-bodied person until 14–16 weeks after their last period. Another procedure is called dilation and evacuation, or D&E. This procedure involves the use of suction as well as medical instruments to empty the uterus. This type of procedure is used if it has been 16 weeks since your last period (each state has different restrictions on how far along they will terminate a pregnancy). In-clinic abortions are close to 100% effective at ending a pregnancy.

In order to complete an abortion, the patient is usually given some pain medicine to help with the discomfort of cramping during the procedure. You may also receive medication that helps your cervix dilate, or open, so that it's easier for the materials inside the uterus to come out. Similar to a pelvic exam, the medical provider will use a speculum to help keep the vagina open so that they can see what they are doing. They then use medical instruments, including a small hand-held suction device, to gently remove the tissue out of the uterus. The entire procedure takes around 5–10 minutes (not counting the prep work and recovery time). After it's completed, you will rest in the recovery room until you're feeling well enough to leave. If you are having an abortion later in the pregnancy, the procedure is a little more involved and you may actually be sedated. Prior to any of these procedures, the medical staff will go over each part of the process so that you're comfortable and know what to expect.

An in-clinic abortion means that you will be experiencing your abortion in the health care facility with doctors, nurses and medical staff on site. Exact protocol for abortions vary from state to state. As with other in-clinic procedures you may have experienced before, upon checking in and prepping for the procedure, the medical staff will go over the details of the procedure and ensure your consent. They will examine you, run some labs and potentially complete an ultrasound to determine how far along you are in the pregnancy, which will ensure proper care. They will also go over how to care for yourself after the procedure is complete. While the procedure is relatively fast, you should plan your abortion to take place when you can take some time off from school and/or work and allow your body to recuperate, as you will likely have cramping and some bleeding for a few days after the procedure. Typically, the cramping and discomfort can be controlled with over-the-counter pain medication like ibuprofen, heating pads, and rest.

Does having an abortion hurt? A lot of people wonder if abortion hurts. Each person's experience is different. Some people feel mild discomfort, while others say it's really painful. This depends on how far along you are in the pregnancy. Medical staff don't want you to be uncomfortable, which is why you get pain medications.

MEDICATION ABORTION

Medication Abortion (or the abortion pill) means that instead of having a procedure, the user takes medicine to end their pregnancy. This option is available to those who are less than eight weeks pregnant. And it's 98–100% effective at ending a pregnancy. If this is the type of abortion you decide to have, you will go to a clinic where a medical provider will give you a pill called mifepristone. This pill is designed to stop the production of progesterone (the hormone your body needs to carry a pregnancy). You will also get a prescription for antibiotics. Then, within six to forty-eight hours of taking the first pill, you take a second pill (at home). This pill is called misoprostal and it is what causes your body to expel the tissue from the uterus. Similar to an in-clinic procedure, you will feel cramping and bleeding as the body expels the tissue from the uterus. Self-care for a medication abortion looks similar to after an in-clinic abortion. It is recommended you take the time for your body to rest, use a heating pad to help with the cramping, and use ibuprofen to help control the pain.

Is abortion safe? Abortion, both in-clinic and medication, is safe. There is little risk involved. Surgical abortion has been done in the U.S. since 1973 and medication abortion has been used in the U.S. for over fifteen years. A medical professional will go over all the risks involved with either the in-clinic procedure or medication abortion prior to having an abortion. If you experience any complications, you will be able to access a twenty-four hour help line to get questions answered and determine if you need further medical care.

Are there any long-term side effects to having an abortion? Short answer: no. There are lots of myths out there about abortion. It's important that you make your decision on fact. Having an abortion does not increase your risk of breast cancer or make it harder to become pregnant later on. Abortion does not mean that you have an increased risk for having a miscarriage or child with a birth defect.

Aren't people who have abortions, well, bad? No. Abortion is a legal medical procedure that, similar to contraception, helps women determine if, how, and when they will have a family. There are many different opinions about abortion out there. And that's okay. Everyone is entitled to their opinion. But there is no reason to feel ashamed or embarrassed if you choose to have an abortion. In fact, one in four women in the United States will have an abortion before they are forty-five years old. [48]

While it's true that only a female-bodied person can become pregnant, they need a male-bodied person to get that way. Therefore, it is necessary for a male-bodied person to recognize their responsibility and the part they play in a pregnancy. If you are a male-bodied person and get a female-bodied person pregnant, it is not just the female-bodied person who is responsible. Both parties' opinions and values should be considered when trying to figure out

---

48 "Considering Abortion." Planned Parenthood. Accessed March 09, 2018. https://www.plannedparenthood.org/learn/abortion/considering-abortion.

the best option for the pregnancy. If parenting is the chosen option, the male-bodied person should take responsibility for the child and support and help raise the child. While, ultimately, the female-bodied person has the right to make the decision regardless of the male-bodied person's wishes, both parties should communicate with each other and work together to find a solution.

CONVERSATION STARTERS . . .

• • • • • • • • • •

The conversation starters are designed to be prompts for having conversations. Feel free to use them in the way that feels right to you.

Questions for Teens to Ask Their Parents

- Abortion laws are different in every state. Why is it easier to access a health service like abortion in some states than in other states?

Questions for Parents to Ask Their Teens

- Did you know that, "The U.S. adolescent pregnancy rate continues to be one of the highest among developed countries. At 43 per 1,000 women aged 15–19 in 2013, it is significantly higher than recent rates found in other developed countries, including France (25 per 1,000) and Sweden (29 per 1,000)."[49] Why do you think this is?

- Together, check out the website: https://www.guttmacher.org/state-policy/explore/overview-abortion-laws. What are the restrictions in your state?

- If you or your partner became pregnant, what options would you consider? Why?

---

49 Sedgh G et al., Adolescent pregnancy, birth, and abortion rates across countries: levels and recent trends, *Journal of Adolescent Health*, 2015, 56(2):223–230.

16

YOU'VE GOTTA TALK ABOUT IT, FOLKS!

It's important that people in all relationships engage in open and honest communication. This is the only way you're going to be able to clearly express your needs and wants and understand those of your partner. When you're engaging in sexual activities, this type of clear communication is crucial. Yeah, yeah. But how do you have open and honest communication?

First of all, communication isn't just talking. There are nonverbal or body clues involved in communication. Like, you know how you can tell your parents are really mad without them saying anything? Sometimes the biggest message can be conveyed in things you don't say. Your gestures, posture, and facial cues all help to emphasize or detract from your message.

There is also listening. Listening and making sure we understand is huge. Sometimes when we are in a conversation, especially when we recognize we don't agree, we may think we are listening when in fact we're thinking about how to

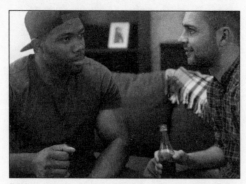

Talking with your partner about sex can be awkward and embarrassing. But if you're comfortable enough to have sex with your partner, shouldn't you be able to talk about it with them? Having open and honest communication about your boundaries, what you like and don't like, and how you want to be treated is really important. Just make sure you have the conversation privately and when you're both giving each other your full attention.

react to what the other person is saying. So, we aren't really listening. You know? In these types of situations, we are not paying attention to all the communication that is happening because we're distracted. In order to really understand a person, we need to focus in on what that person is saying, all of what they are saying (verbally and non-verbally). If we don't actively listen we might as well not be communicating with each other because the communication is lost. Listening is just as important as the message that is being given.

EFFECTIVE COMMUNICATION

In order to understand how to effectively communicate, you need to understand that the most effective communication is open and honest. But what does that look like? Let's break it down. First, you need to set the scene. As in, where and when is this communication going to happen? Think about when your message is going to be received well, like when you will have your partner's undivided attention. Usually, this is before you get into certain situations. (Those situations where you really need to communicate your boundaries. Probably not the best to discuss those boundaries as you're getting busy, you know?) Let's say you really like a person and are alone with them. You want to communicate your boundaries (what you are and are not willing to do sexually) before you start to get into it. By telling your partner what you do and don't want to

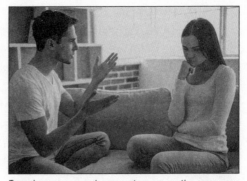

To make sure you and your partner are on the same page when it comes to sex, make sure you talk about it before you get into a sexual situation.

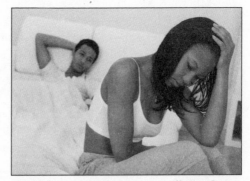

Nonverbal communication can be very effective. Be sure to pay attention to your partner's nonverbal clues like body position and eye contact. Having open and honest communication takes practice and can sometimes feel scary. But it builds a foundation of trust between partners that enhances the relationship and helps make sex great when you and your partner decide you're ready.

do before getting sexual, you will find you're more successful in sticking with your limits. The timing for communication is really important. If one of you is distracted, the message you're trying to convey may not be heard or received well.

227

Talking face-to-face is going to be best, especially if it's a challenging subject. I know what you're thinking: "Why? Can't I just take the easy way out and text what I want to say?" True, it's often easier to "talk" about difficult things when you aren't face-to-face, especially if you think the other person is going to be bummed or angry by what you have to say. But, the problem with texting or email or even the phone is that you can't see the other person. You can't see their physical or nonverbal clues. You can't be sure that they understand what you're trying to convey.

> **HELPFUL HINT:** Practice·make perfect! Write down what you want to say prior to saying it to the person, especially if you think the conversation is going to be difficult. This way you can focus on the conversation and not worry about whether you've made all the points you want to make.

Effective communication also means that you're practicing honest communication. Being transparent about why you do or don't want to do something sexually helps people understand and support your decisions. So, for example, if you decide you don't want to have sex without a condom because neither you nor your partner have been tested for STIs, say it. (Then go get tested!) Or, if you make a mistake, own it and apologize. No one is perfect or right all the time.

Effective communication means listening and checking to make sure what you heard is correct. Sometimes this means repeating what they say back to them, to make sure you've understood. Other times it means asking questions to clarify. You can only be responsible for your own communication. If your partner or friend isn't committed to communicating openly and honestly, and they interpret your communication differently than you intended without checking, that's on them. You can only do your best.

Nonverbal communication (or body language and facial expressions) is a big part of making sure your message is understood. Make sure what you're saying matches what your body is saying. If it doesn't, it's easy for the recipient of the message to be confused. If you don't want to do something, use a firm voice, say a clear "No," and make sure your body matches that. So, cross your arms (which shows a closed-off body) or shake your head. Make sure your nonverbal communication matches your verbal communication, as that's the best way to make sure your message is heard.

> Typically, in a sexual situation, a person's body physically reacts. For example, a female-bodied person may have increased discharge, or feel "wet," after kissing and heavy petting. Or a male-bodied person's penis may become erect. This is totally normal and makes sense because the body is being sexually stimulated. Just because a person's body is having this reaction, though, it does not mean they want to have sex or should have sex. It's just the body's physiological reaction, and it does not necessarily reflect what a person should do or wants to do.

Own your decisions and what you want to say. Try to use "I" statements as much as you can. For example, "I don't want to have sex until we both get tested for STIs." Instead of, "You need to get tested before we have sex." Again, own it. When you say "you" instead of "I" it can be interpreted as attacking the other person. And when someone feels attacked, they go into defense mode. They stop listening and are only thinking of how to defend themselves.

Speak up and advocate for yourself. Dropping clues or hints is not open and honest communication. Your partner isn't a mind reader. If you want things to be a certain way, say it. If you're upset or angry about something, tell them. Your actions or behavior might tell them that you're mad, but they won't know what about until you say it.

> Good communication is sexy! When you're ready to have sex, good communication is what is going to make it good. That's right. The difference between "good sex" and "bad sex"? Talking about it. Just think about it. If you can honestly tell your partner what you like and don't like, they'll know. And if they know, they can do the things you like. And then sex can be really good. Like, really good. So, if you aren't ready to tell your partner what you want to do sexually, or you aren't willing to hear that from them, then you might not be ready to have sex. Think about it. Sex is supposed to feel good. How can it if you don't communicate about it?

That brings us to communication when you are fighting or angry with a person. When you're angry, it's really hard to practice open and honest communication that is respectful of the person or people you're mad at. And everyone gets mad at something. So how do you make sure that you have the opportunity to be angry and disagree with a person while still being respectful?

Stop and take a break

If you're really angry—like, want to scream angry—stop what you're doing, take a step back and breathe. Maybe even remove yourself from the situation. Give yourself time to cool off by taking a walk, going into another room, listening to music, or doing whatever you can to give yourself some distance from the person and situation. Relax and calm down. Giving yourself (and the other person or people) some time can help to keep the situation from escalating or getting worse.

Think about the situation

Once you've calmed down, think about what happened to make you so mad. Was it something the other person said? Something they did? Is that really what happened, or what you interpreted it to be? Maybe you have been holding onto anger about something completely unassociated with this event. Are you really angry about that last little trigger? Or has your anger been building up over time? Figure out what really made you mad, and then address it with the person (or people).

Talk about it

After you've figured out what you are upset about, explain it to the other person. Use "I" statements when you can, and make sure they understand what you're saying by checking for understanding. Before you start talking, though, make sure the other person is ready and calmed down as well. If they aren't ready, give them more time. If you try to have a conversation when they are still mad, even if you're calm, you're going to be right back where you were: fighting. It's okay if you don't resolve an issue right away. It's okay to give both of you the time you need to think about what's going on and what you want. By giving yourself and the other person this space, you can be sure that when you do talk, you are actively listening and problem solving.

Listen to the other person

Once you tell the other person (or people) how you feel, listen to what they have to say. No, really listen. Don't just think about what you want to say next, but listen to their side of things. Always check for understanding and whether what you heard is actually what they were trying to say.

If needed, apologize or accept an apology. If you aren't ready to accept the apology or to apologize, then give yourself some more time. Just remember, if you accept an apology, then you have to let the issue rest. You don't get to hold onto it for ammunition to use in a later disagreement. (If this is something you're doing or you find a friend or partner is doing to you, keep that in mind when you read over the information on healthy relationships starting on page 245.)

Being open and honest with your communication isn't easy and takes lots of practice. The more you do it, the better you will get at it. Just remember that no one is perfect and we all make mistakes in our communication. Learn from those mistakes and move on. Another key thing to remember in open and honest communication is that you only have control over how you communicate. If the other person interprets what you say and doesn't check for understanding, that's on them. You can only control your side of the communication and do your best.

Communication and Consent

So obviously communicating about what you do and don't want to do sexually also means asking for permission to engage in sexual activity. It also means respecting your partner's boundaries and not coercing them into doing something they don't want to do. Following the guidelines for open and honest communication will help with having the conversation with your partner about sex and boundaries.

Before kissing or touching another person, you need to ask them if it's okay. Yep. You literally need to say, "is it okay if I kiss you?" or "Can I kiss you?" That's clear communication. Then, the other person knows what you're asking and can tell you "yes" or "no." And if it's "no," then you don't do it. Full stop. You don't get to beg or try to convince them that it will be fun. It was a "no." Listen to it and move on.

You might think that it isn't romantic or sexy to ask a person for their consent to kiss them. Wrong! In fact, getting and giving consent is super sexy. Because you know that both of you are into it (and into each other), and that feels pretty great.

SOME IDEAS ABOUT HOW TO ASK FOR CONSENT:

"Would you like it if I...?"

"I really like it when..."

"Do feel like you're ready for...?"

"What do you think about trying...?"

SOME IDEAS ABOUT
HOW TO GIVE CONSENT:

"Yes!"

"I would like to try..."

"It really feels good when you..."

"I really like..."

Things to remember about consent:

Consent is always freely given. If someone is drunk, high, or passed out, they can't give consent.

Just because you consent to a behavior once does not mean that you give consent to that behavior every time. In fact, you may say "yes" to something and then change your mind while you're doing that something. That's okay. And your partner needs to respect that and stop the behavior.

Make sure you completely understand what you're giving consent to. Giving consent to being walked home by a person from a party does not mean that you're giving consent to have them over for sex. Those are two totally different things.

Giving consent should feel good and be something that you're excited about. This is about engaging in sexual behaviors that you *and* your partner want to do. If you're not excited about it, or your partner isn't excited about it, stop what you're doing and check in. Is this really what you both want?

It's important to know that there are laws about consent. These vary from state to state and have to do with age, whether someone is drunk, high, or passed out, or whether a person is disabled. To understand the laws in each state and to understand where you can get help if you have been the victim of sexual assault, please check out the RAINN (Rape, Abuse & Incest National Network) organization. It's a national organization that can provide support to victims of sexual assault 24/7 online and by phone. The website is www.rainn.org, and the free hotline is 1-800-656-HOPE.

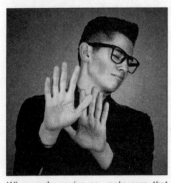

When you're saying no, make sure that what you're saying is matched with clear body language. Obviously, this person is a bit dramatic, but sometimes, when you want to make sure your message is heard, being dramatic isn't a bad thing!

Saying "No" and Listening to "No"

While there may be things that you're okay with doing sexually, there may be other things you aren't ready for, or things that are just nonstarters. Like, you know you never want to do x, y, or z. And while everyone should be able to hear a "no" message no matter what that looks like, it will help if you're very clear in giving that "no" message.

So, how do you make your "no" clear?

First, you can just say the word "no." Use a clear verbal "no" along with clear body language. Other ways to say no are:

- "I don't like that."

- "I don't want to do that."

- "I'm not ready for that."

- "I really like you, but don't want to do that."

- "I'd like to stop."

- "I thought I wanted to, but I changed my mind and I don't want to."

- "Stop."

Clear body language might involve just a shake of the head. It might also involve you needing to physically separate yourself from the other person. If your body language doesn't match what you're saying, the other person is going to be confused. Make sure you are assertive in your

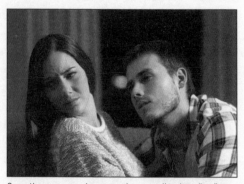

Sometimes, even when you give a really clear "no," your partner tries to convince you to say "yes." Your partner should respect your "no" response regardless of what they want. It takes two to have sex. If one partner doesn't want to, it's a no-go. A partner saying "no" isn't code for "convince me." It's straight-up "no." No means no. And P.S., it doesn't matter if you and your partner have had sex before. If one of you isn't into it? Then it isn't going to happen.

"no" and that it is loud enough for the other person to hear. Sometimes, it helps to suggest an alternative action you are willing to do, like go to the movies.

So, what if you're already participating in a sexual activity and you'd like to stop? Or what if your partner is starting to engage in an activity that makes you uncomfortable, and they haven't asked if they could? Or what if you thought you wanted to do something and you started to do it, but then changed your mind? You still have a right to say "no" and to expect that your partner will listen. Make sure you use both your "no" message and clear body language—in other words, make sure you stop doing the sexual behavior too and distance yourself from your partner. You have the right to say "no" to a sexual behavior at any point. Period. No matter what, you can say "no."

If you hear a "no," listen! You don't get to try to coerce (force or convince against their will) the other person into doing what you want them to do. Listening doesn't just mean hearing a firm "no." Pay attention to the other person's body language. If their "yes" seems timid or unsure, or worried, ask again. Chances are they are not freely consenting. Check in with the person during the behavior. For example, "Does that feel good to you?" Or "Would you like me to (fill in the blank)?" If a person responds with "I don't know," or they don't say anything, guess what? They aren't consenting. Stop what's going on and talk about it. And again, just because they said yes to something yesterday or a week ago, or an hour ago, doesn't mean they have given you permission to do that behavior every time.

Think about if you want to borrow your friend's car. You ask your friend to borrow the car. They will likely ask you where you're driving it to and whether you can fill it up with gas. If you agree, you have their consent to use their car that one time, for that one thing. You wouldn't assume you could just use their car whenever and for whatever. You would ask them each and every time. And, because it is their car, they get to decide whether they want you to use it. They will make that decision based on their needs and desires and feelings.

Oh, and P.S., you know those gender roles we talked about in chapter 9? It's not up to a female identifying person to say "no" or for a male identifying person to initiate sexual behaviors. Consent, both giving and receiving, is for all genders and all types of relationships.

It's *never* okay for someone to touch you in a sexual way without your permission. And if someone does, *it is not your fault*. Remember, you can only control your communication and behavior. It doesn't matter what you're wearing or where you are. No matter what, if you're forced to do something sexual that you don't want to do, the other person is responsible.

> Remember, if a person does not give consent for sex and you engage in the behavior anyway, you are committing sexual assault, which is illegal.

- If you decide you want to dress sexy, that is not an invitation for sex.

- If you flirt with another person, that is not an invitation for sex.

- If you decide you want to be alone with someone, that is not an invitation for sex.

- If you decide to go for a walk, at night, by yourself, that is not an invitation for sex.

If you're feeling pressured or guilty about saying "no," and/or your partner makes you feel bad about saying "no," and/or they react negatively (like sad or mad) when you say no, and/or they completely ignore your "no," it could be that your partner doesn't respect consent. These are all red flags and should be considered as warnings for an unhealthy relationship. Relationships are discussed in chapter 17.

Important note for parents—if your teen is under the age of 18 and they tell you about a sexual assault you may be obligated to report the sexual assault to the authorities. Here's a great resource to become familiar with the laws in your state: www.ageofconsentlaws.net.

Talking to your teen about consent can be triggering if you are survivor of sexual assault. Here's a great place to get support: www.aftersilence.org.

Here's another great resource if you think your teen or someone they know has been sexually assaulted: www.rainn.org.

LET'S PRACTICE!

It might seem a little corny, but thinking about what you want to have happen before you get into certain situations can help you be more successful in achieving your goals. These are some possible situations. If you want, you can talk them out with your parents, or you can go through them on your own. Feel free to write down what you might do or just talk it out.

Let's pretend that you and the person you have a crush on are at a party. Your crush asks you to go upstairs to the bedroom so that the two of you can talk by yourselves. You're excited and flattered that your crush asked you to go upstairs, but you're also nervous about being alone with them because, while you're attracted to them and want them to like you, you aren't ready to do anything more than kiss the person.

- What could you do before going upstairs to make sure you aren't in a situation that might be uncomfortable?

- Even though you told your crush before you went upstairs that you're okay with just talking, your crush starts to kiss you. What is something you could do or say to make sure it doesn't go any further?

- You and your crush have been kissing for a while and they start to touch you on your genitals. While it feels good, you aren't ready. How could you tell your crush? What are some things you could do nonverbally to make sure they hear you aren't ready?

Okay, new situation. Let's pretend that you and your partner are trying to figure out how to "take your relationship to the next level." Meaning, you have decided you're both ready for sex (this could be oral, anal, or vaginal). What are some things you might say to your partner?

- How would you do it? Like, where would you have the conversation?

- How would you know your partner is cool with what you want to do?

MAKING SENSE OF "IT"

- What if they aren't cool with it? How could you respond respectfully?

Okay, final situation. You and your partner (who are both in high school) have gone out on a couple of dates (or hung out together a few times). You've kissed and held hands, and you know that you aren't ready for sex yet. In fact, you're committed to not having sex until you have graduated high school. How and when do you think you should tell your partner?

CONVERSATION STARTERS . . .

• • • • • • • • • •

The conversation starters are designed to be prompts for having conversations. Feel free to use them in the way that feels right to you.

Questions for Teens to Ask Their Parents

- What do you think the easiest thing about effective communication is?

- Do you think we (the parent and the teen) have positive communication? If yes, what do you think we do well? If no, what could we do a better job of?

- What are your experiences asking for consent? Do you think it is hard or easy? Why?

- Have you ever had to say "no" to someone? What did you do that was effective?

- Can you think of a time where you thought you were being clear with your communication and realized that you weren't? What happened? What do you think would have made it more effective?

Questions for Parents to Ask Their Teens*

- Do you think we (the parent and the teen) have good communication? Why or why not?

- If you think we do have good communication, what do you think we do well?

- What do you think we can work to improve when it comes to communication?

- (If your teen has a partner) How would you describe your communication with your partner?

- What experiences have you had asking for consent or giving consent (doesn't have to be a sexual situation)?

- What are some things you could say to your partner to make sure that they respect and honor your communication?

- What do you think is hard about talking to your partner about sex or sexual things? What are some things that might make it easier?

*Be aware that education and discussions around consent may lead to a disclosure about abuse or sexual assault (either from your teen or a disclosure about a friend or acquaintance of the teen). Before entering into a conversation about consent, please refresh yourself with the suggestions in chapter 16 about how to be supportive and provide helpful non-judgmental support.

17

WHAT HEALTHY RELATIONSHIPS LOOK LIKE . . .

There are all sorts of relationships out there. Think of all the relationships you're in. You have relationships with your parents, friends, other family members, and if you don't already, you will likely have a romantic relationship at some point. All of these relationships are either "healthy," as in they make you feel good, and you and the other person get positive things out of it, or "unhealthy." Simply put, healthy relationships make you feel good and unhealthy relationships make you feel bad. You might feel bad about yourself, or anxious about being around the person. But relationships are complicated. Some of them can make you feel both good and bad, and it isn't always easy to figure out whether a relationship is healthy or unhealthy. And if it's unhealthy, it isn't always easy to get out of that relationship.

HEALTHY RELATIONSHIPS
A healthy relationship means that you have respect for the other person and the other person has respect for you.

Respect means that you value each other, listen to each other, compromise, help each other, and treat the other person like you want to be treated. A healthy relationship means that both of you are equally

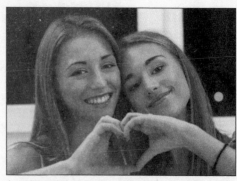

A healthy relationship is built on trust and respect. Trust and respect need to be built and that can take time. It can also mean making yourself vulnerable and that can be scary. Having a healthy relationship isn't easy, it takes a lot of hard work. But that hard work is worth it to have a loving relationship.

invested in the relationship. It doesn't mean you don't fight, but it depends on how you fight. Do you listen to one another's points? Really listen and not just try to think of what you're going to say in return? Do you both make compromises? Do you forgive each other and not hold a grudge? Fighting is totally normal in a relationship and fights are never fun, but if you and your partner have a healthy relationship, you will both grow from the disagreement and you will both work to see each other's point of view, forgive each other, and talk things out calmly and respectfully. People involved in a healthy relationship don't hit each other when they fight. They do not disrespect each other by calling each other names or putting each other down.

Respect in a romantic relationship also means that each of you recognizes that you both have valid feelings and can have different needs, and that those needs are equally important and valued. It means that when you need space or time apart, you get it (and give it). A healthy romantic relationship means that you support each other and build each other up, not tear each other down. A healthy relationship is one where you respect and honor each other's boundaries, including sexual boundaries.

A healthy relationship is also one in which you and your partner trust each other. But what does that mean, to trust someone? Well, do you feel safe with the person? Do you feel like they believe in you (and you believe in them)? Keep in mind, relationships don't instantly have trust. Trust is something that is built over time. Sure, you might have a gut instinct that you can trust a person (and often that gut instinct is right on), but trust is built over time. In order to say you're in a trusting relationship, it must be something that both of you feel and are invested in.

When you're thinking about your relationship and trying to assess whether there is a foundation of trust, think about whether or not you feel heard and supported. Is your partner there for you? Maybe not physically, but emotionally? Do they have your back? What about you? Are you there for them? Do you support your partner? If your relationship is healthy then you can rely on them to be a safe and supportive person no matter what.

Building trust can happen by talking (and listening) to each other. It is linked to respect, because you can respect each other's points of views and trust that, the other person won't judge you or belittle you for your views. Trust is developed after going through various experiences together and demonstrating your respect in various situations. If there isn't trust in a relationship, partners can feel insecure and/ or jealous. Sure, these types of feelings are pretty normal to have, even in a healthy relationship. But be wary, if that jealousy or insecurity is pervasive, or it starts to impact how you relate to one another, that can be a warning sign that something unhealthy is happening.

In order to build trust in a relationship, you and your partner need to be honest with each other. Honesty means that you tell each other the truth. You tell them what you like and don't like in a respectful way. You're up front about things, you don't make your partner guess. While telling the truth can be intimidating and scary, it shouldn't be something you're afraid of. You shouldn't fear that your partner will hurt you or make you feel like less of a person. If you tell the truth and your partner isn't receptive (as in they react violently or become emotionally of mentally abusive) don't ignore that red flag as it could mean that your relationship isn't healthy.

Honesty also means that you admit when you're wrong or make a mistake and know that your partner will forgive you (not hold it against you for later). I know, it's hard to admit when you're wrong or make a mistake. But if you don't own it with your partner, it's going to mean that your relationship isn't built on honesty, and it will erode the trust in your relationship. No one is right all the time (even though we would like to be). Be humble enough to admit it.

Another foundation of a healthy relationship is equality. Both you and your partner should be showing up equally to the relationship. It should be 50/50. Sure, that balance might shift if one of you is going through a rough patch and needs a little extra support, but in order to have a healthy relationship, both of you need to come to it equally.

Decisions should be made with both of you providing input. This goes for decisions that are small, like where you're going to eat or what movie you're going to see, or bigger decisions, like those that involve sex. Is it okay if your partner wants to surprise you with a date they planned? Of course! But there are times when surprises aren't okay—like when it comes to being sexual. Defining what you're going to do together sexually is for both of you to decide—equally. Remember consent? (Check out chapter 16 for a refresher.) Same goes for contraception and STI transmission prevention. You and your partner need to come to a decision together on what method(s) you're going to use. You are both equally at risk, so take on the responsibility together. Additionally, people in healthy relationships know how to compromise and live with that compromise.

Not all of these things are easy. In fact, they can be really hard. Good communication is critical. You have to be able to talk about, well, all the things. A healthy relationship is one where you can talk about your feelings and work through disagreements. Especially when it comes to boundaries and sex. You might be ready to do one thing sexually but your partner isn't. In a healthy relationship, you might be upset or disappointed that you aren't both ready to do the same things, but you respect that you are at different places with regards to sex and together work to find a compromise—something you're both comfortable doing. People in a healthy relationship don't guilt their partner or make them feel bad (or force them) to do something sexually if they aren't ready.

Suggestions to Make Your Relationship Great

- Be confident in who you are. You are great. Truly. Show yourself some love. When you love yourself, you are able to be a better partner to another person.

- Help your partner know how great they are (and expect your partner to do the same for you). Seriously, you really like each other, right? Let them know!

- Talk about sex. Talk about what you like, what you don't like, how you're going to stay safe, and what your boundaries are.

- Listen to each other. Especially when you're expressing your feelings. They are both important and valid.

- Be honest with each other.

- Don't be afraid to spend time apart and have independent activities and friends. In fact, this can bring some diversity to the relationship and make it exciting and interesting.

- Forgive each other.

Unhealthy Relationships

You're in an unhealthy relationship if you're not being respected, or if you are being physically or mentally abused. No one tries to start an unhealthy relationship. Why would they? If the person you were thinking of getting into a relationship with treated you badly at the start of the relationship, why would you get into a relationship with them?

The lack of respect and poor treatment typically starts very slowly and usually in a way you might not notice, or would easily forgive. It might also begin with you second-guessing whether "it was really that bad" (whatever "it" might be). Likely your partner will be immediately remorseful or feel bad about what happened and assure you that it will never happen again. It might even feel good that someone could get that passionate about you or that jealous or upset over something that involves you! And if this happens on occasion, it's probably not an unhealthy relationship—no relationship is perfect. But if you see this as a repeated pattern and it happens in conjunction with some of the following behaviors, you want to talk to you parents and friends about it—they can help you figure out what to do.

Unhealthy relationships are often also referred to as abusive relationships. But don't get hung up on the vocabulary; think about how the relationship makes you feel. If you don't feel good about yourself when you're with the other person, it probably isn't healthy. Abuse is often thought of as something physical that happens, and being physically hurt is never okay. If you have been or are being physically hurt by your partner, get help. But abuse isn't always physical. It can be mental and emotional.

Emotional and mental abuse can be much harder to pick up on because they are often subtler. This type of abuse can show itself in many ways. You know how we talked about it kind of feeling good when a partner gets jealous? Well, that can be taken too far. Like if a partner doesn't want you to spend time with anyone else because they only want you to be with them. Or they need you to be there for them all the time. You turn into their only source of, well, anything. Like, if you want to break up, they threaten to kill themselves or, if you want to go out with your friends (without them), they say that you have ruined their night because they won't have any fun without you.

Someone who is emotionally or mentally abusive will also belittle you and your feelings. Saying things like, "you're just too sensitive!" or, when something is going wrong, you "just need to get over it!" If it was a healthy relationship, your partner would support your feelings and help you process them, not make you put them aside or say they don't matter.

We already talked a little bit about the fact that a partner who is controlling might demand all your time, but they will also want to check your phone, know who you're talking to via phone or text, question where you are, and check up on you to make sure you're where you say you are.

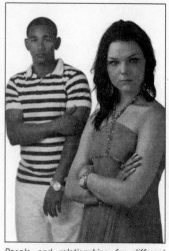

People end relationships for different reasons. Sometimes, it's due to trust being broken. Sometimes, it's because someone doesn't feel like they are being respected. As you develop as an individual, the things you want and need in a partner can change. That's totally normal. So sometimes, one or both people in the relationship figure out it's just not working. When that happens, it's best to end the relationship as soon as you can even though it's really hard.

Another sign of an unhealthy relationship is that you'll find that your partner is slowly changing who you are. For example, if your partner doesn't like your friends, you may find that you stop seeing your friends. Or maybe you have always played basketball and now that you're with this person you stop playing because they say it takes too much time away from them. Remember, if it's a healthy relationship, your partner will celebrate and support your interests, not make you stop being who you are.

Finally, if you're in an unhealthy relationship, you may find that your goals in life begin to change. If you want to go out for an activity at school, your partner should be encouraging you and helping you achieve your goals. An unhealthy relationship will put you down, tell you that you shouldn't try, and basically try to control what you do through what seems like advice but is really unhealthy manipulation.

Like I said, one or two of these behaviors, on occasion, is probably okay. People are human, after all, and learning how to be in a relationship takes work. But if you're seeing a pattern or your friends or parents bring it to your attention that they think you are changing or are worried about you, pay attention. You might want to think about ending the relationship. Often people think they can change the person or that the situation will get better on its own. It won't, and they won't change unless they recognize there is a problem and they make the decision to change. For more information on how to get help with an abusive relationship, go to: http://www.loveisrespect.org/. Remember, it's *not your fault*. You do *not* deserve to be treated badly. No one does.

Not sure what type of relationship you're in? Check out www.loveisrepect.org/#quizhome for online quizzes that help you assess whether your relationship is healthy or unhealthy and to find out if you're a good partner.

Ending a Relationship

Typically, when you enter a relationship, you aren't thinking about how you're going to end it. But if a romantic relationship does end, it's hard. Whether the relationship has been healthy or unhealthy, ending a relationship is never fun because you did, or still do, care about the other person. And just because the romantic relationship ends, it doesn't mean the feelings you have for another person always go away.

People end relationships for lots of different reasons. Maybe they aren't in love any more. Maybe they don't want to be in a relationship. Maybe they need to focus on their schoolwork. Or maybe the relationship is unhealthy. If the relationship was healthy but you're moving on, how you approach a breakup looks different than it does when you're ending an unhealthy relationship. Whatever the reason, remember to practice your healthy communication skills.

Ending a relationship that has been healthy

If you're the one who wants to end the relationship, be honest with your partner. Don't string them along. Don't be mean. Be honest and considerate. Get together (yeah, in person) and explain that you do not want to be in a relationship anymore and why. Don't break up over the phone or via text or email. Sure, this might feel easier, but remember, you liked this person. You respect this person. Show them that same respect when you're ending the relationship. (I never said this was going to be pleasant or easy.)

Here are some ideas for how to end a romantic relationship:

- "I've really had a good time with you, but I don't want to be in a relationship right now so I think we should break up."

- "I think we should break up. I've met another person that I like, and it isn't fair to you for us to stay together when I am not 100% into it."

- "I think we should break up. I'm not ready for a committed and serious relationship."

After the Breakup
It's normal to feel sad or even angry after a relationship ends (even if you were the one who ended it). Sometimes, you just need to be in that sadness for a minute and watch the sappy movie and eat the tub of ice cream. But you can't stay in that funk. There are lots of people out there! Sure, the person you were dating probably had become a big part of your life and you probably spent a lot of time together so it's normal to feel lonely after a break up. Try to surround yourself with friends and family. Force yourself to get off the couch and go do things. Is there a hobby or class or activity you have been thinking about trying? Go do it! This is a great time to try something new. This feeling won't last forever.

Ending a relationship that has been unhealthy
If you're getting out of an unhealthy relationship, it's still normal to miss your partner. Just because your partner was a jerk doesn't mean they don't have any good qualities. (Otherwise you wouldn't have started dating them in the first place!)

It can be helpful to write a list of the ways they have treated you poorly so that you can remind yourself why you aren't together if you start feeling like you want to get back together. Because your partner likely isolated you or made decisions for you, being faced with loneliness and decision making might feel a bit overwhelming. This is normal. Make sure your support system (parents, family, friends, school, counselor, whomever) knows what is going on and don't hesitate to reach out to them for help. That's what they are there for!

I have different suggestions for ending an unhealthy relationship than if it's healthy. First of all, because it's unhealthy, you can expect that your partner will use some of the controlling methods that they used when you were together, like threatening to kill themselves or making you feel guilty. For this reason, think about breaking up with the person while a family member or friend is with you. Or, if you feel like it might become physically unsafe, consider breaking up over the phone or via email. Say what you need to say and that's it. Your partner will likely be mad or try to twist your words around. Just say what you need to say and leave. There is nothing you can say that will make your partner happy. Trust yourself and trust your gut. If you're feeling afraid, you probably have a good reason for it.

After the break up, make sure you are safe—if they come to the door, don't answer it. Make sure people know you aren't together anymore so they can help get your back. It's okay to tell the school what is going on so they can alert security if they need to. Always keep a cell phone with you so you can call someone (or even 911) if you need help and avoid isolated areas and being alone. If your ex threatens you, tell someone! If they send texts or emails or post threats online, save them and show them to your parents and even the police. If you're in immediate danger, call 911.

For more help with ending an abusive relationship go to: www.loveisrespect.org. They have counselors you can talk to 24/7 and they can help you figure out how to stay safe in your particular situation. They also have an online interactive safety plan to help you get out of your relationship.

What do you think?

Go through the following situations with your parents and talk them out. See if you think what is being described is a healthy or unhealthy relationship. Do you and your parent agree or disagree?

Situation #1:
When you go out without your partner, they ask you to call or text them when you get home. When you do, they ask you what you did and who you did it with. You share what you did and with whom, and then they ask you if you want to hang out the next day. You can't, even though it's Saturday, because you're going to your aunt's for dinner and have a big test you need to study for. Your partner is upset because they aren't going to be able to hang out with you. They tell you that you aren't making enough time for them. You apologize and tell them you will be able to get a cup of coffee with them on Sunday, and they reluctantly agree to going with you for coffee. Is this a healthy relationship or an unhealthy relationship? Why do you think that?

Answer:
This is a healthy relationship. It's normal to miss spending time with someone you really like (like your partner). You're both forgiving and willing to compromise. They are concerned with your safety and supportive of your time apart.

257

Situation #2:

You stayed late at basketball practice, and when you come out of the locker room, your partner is waiting for you in the parking lot. You're surprised because you didn't know they would be waiting for you. As you get into their car and say hello, your partner doesn't answer and gives you the silent treatment. After a couple of minutes, they pull the car over and yell, "Why were you so late?" As you explain that you stayed late at practice to get some one-on-one coaching on your jump shot, your partner sinisterly says, "Yeah, I know. You wanted extra one-on-one time with the coach. Because you have a crush on them, don't you?" You deny the crush and try to get them calmed down, but they won't let it go. In order to try to make things better, you offer your phone to your partner and tell them they can look through your contacts, calls, and text history. This calms your partner down but they won't drive you home until they have gone through your whole phone. After 20 minutes, and a call from your parent, they finally drive you home. Is this a healthy or unhealthy relationship? Why do you think that?

Answer:

This is definitely something you should pay attention to—it may be a sign of an unhealthy relationship. Could it be a one-time thing? Possibly. But the combination of behaviors should definitely make you be cautious. Regardless of the fact that you're late, you do not deserve to be yelled at. Also, you have the right to privacy. While you offered up your phone, they should be able to trust you without proof.

Situation #3:

You and your partner are making out and the two of you are moving pretty fast sexually. You've never talked about having sex before and you want to stop because you aren't sure you are ready. You tell your partner you want to stop and they do, but they are frustrated and tell you they thought they were going to have sex tonight. They thought you were "good to go." As you explain that you aren't ready because you haven't talked about protection and haven't gotten tested for STIs yet, your partner agrees that you haven't talked about it and, while they are disappointed, they understand how you feel. Then they ask you what you're willing to do since they are already sexually aroused. When you explain that you aren't willing to do anything else, they try to convince you to change your mind. When you stay strong and repeat that you aren't ready, they finally stop asking and give you your space. They are a little mad, but eventually let it go. Is this a healthy or unhealthy relationship? Why do you think that?

Answer:

This is a healthy relationship. Sure, it would have been ideal for you two to talk about sex before getting into the situation, but your partner still respected your boundaries. While they were mad and frustrated, they were able to move on and still enjoy being with you.

Situation #4:

You and your partner have been seeing each other exclusively for a couple of months and they are super nice to you. They buy you presents, take you out to eat and encourage you in school. Since you two have been dating, you don't see your friends very often. In fact, your best friend stops you in school and tells you that they miss hanging out. You realize that you've been spending all your time on school-work and with your partner, and decide to make plans with your best friend to hang out on Friday night. When you tell your partner, they say, "What the hell? Why do you want to hang out with them? They're a terrible influence! All you need in your life is me. Your friends will only drag you down. How could you be so stupid?" Is this a healthy or unhealthy relationship? Why do you think that?

Answer:
This is an unhealthy relationship. Remember, each of you are entitled to have friends outside of the relationship and be an independent person outside of the relationship. Additionally, people in healthy relationships do not call each other names and put each other down.

CONVERSATION STARTERS . . .

• • • • • • • • • •

The conversation starters are designed to be prompts for having conversations. Feel free to use them in the way that feels right to you.

Questions for Teens to Ask Their Parents

• What do you think is the best part about being in a relationship?

• What do you think is the hardest thing about being in a relationship?

• Have you ever had to break up with someone?

• If yes, how did it happen? Looking back, would you do anything differently? How did you feel? Why?

• Has anyone ever broken up with you? How did you feel? Why? What would have made it better?

• What are some things you do to help you feel better when you're sad or upset? What advice would you give a friend who has just broken up with their partner?

• When you decided you were ready to have sex, did you talk to your partner about it ahead of time? If yes, was it easy or hard? What made it easy/what made it hard? If no, why not? Do you wish you had talked about it?

• When you think about the first time you had sex, would you do anything differently?

- Have you ever had an unhealthy relationship? If yes, how did you know that it was unhealthy? What did you do to take care of yourself?

Questions for Parents to Ask Their Teens

- Are you in a relationship? If yes:

  a.) Do you feel like your partner listens to you and respects you?

  b.) Have you talked about sex and whether you're going to be sexually active? Have you talked about how to stay safe?

  c.) Do you feel supported by your partner?

- Have you ever broken up with someone or been broken up with? If yes, how did you feel? What helped you feel better? If no, do you want to end a relationship and do you need help?

- What are some things you're looking for in a relationship? (If they are currently in a relationship) Do you feel like you have those things in your relationship? If not, what's missing? Are those things deal breakers (as in you shouldn't be together anymore)?

- Are any of your friends dating? If yes, what do you think about their relationships? If no, why do you think that is?

- What do you think is the hardest part about being in a relationship?

- What is one thing you're nervous about or think will be difficult to navigate in a relationship?

18

STAYING SAFE: UNDERSTANDING SEXUAL HARASSMENT AND ASSAULT, INCLUDING HOW TO GET HELP AND HOW TO BE AN ACTIVE BYSTANDER
(TRIGGER WARNING)

In this section, I am using female and male or woman and man instead of female-bodied or male-bodied. It's more common for a person to be sexually violated and objectified based on how the aggressor interprets their identity, not necessarily based on biological sex.

We talked a lot about consent in chapter 16. We've also spent a lot of time talking about healthy relationships and setting boundaries. But no matter how safe you are, you may find yourself sexually violated. Sexual violations run a wide spectrum, all the way from verbal statements to the act of rape. Regardless of the violation, they leave the survivor feeling violated and emotionally traumatized. Every person who has been violated in this way has a different reaction. Every person who has experienced a sexual violation processes it and incorporates it into their life in different ways. There is no one right way to react, process, or deal with a sexual violation.

As I mentioned, there are, unfortunately, different ways a person can be sexually assaulted. Some cases of sexual assault and harassment are very easy to understand and are clearly defined in law. Rape, child pornography, human trafficking—these are all very serious crimes that are clearly defined and as a result, can more easily be prosecuted. Other situations aren't as easily defined or documented. Also, there is a lot of victim-blaming that happens when it comes to harassment and assault, as well as an established track record of criminals not being prosecuted or getting lenient sentences.

While some violations are very definitive, others are not considered illegal, like getting whistled at by someone in a passing car. This is a violation, or harassment. It's something that happens all the time. My guess is that the person who did the whistling wasn't thinking, "I want to violate that person." Maybe they were, but likely they were thinking, *whoa! That person is really attractive and I want them to know!* This attention was not asked for (no matter what the person is wearing, looks like, or is doing) and their body is being objectified. When we are talking about sexual violations and harassment, it's not necessarily about the intention of the person who is making the comments or committing the violation, but how the targeted person, or person who is the recipient of the aggression, feels and interprets what was done. If the person who was whistled at feels harassed or violated, then they were.

Bottom line is if you have been victimized, it can be hard to feel supported and find justice. A great resource is the National Sexual Assault Hotline. The number is 1-800-656-HOPE. This organization can assist with both assault and harassment. If you don't want to call, you can also go online to www.rainn.org to chat with someone and/or find additional resources. Another good resource to understand your rights, especially when it comes to sexual harassment and discrimination in a school setting, is the United States Department of Education Office for Civil Rights at www2. ed.gov/about/offices/list/ocr/index.html. General information about laws specific to your state can be found at www. americanbar.org/groups/women/resources/discrimination. html. This website has an interactive map and additional resources about bullying (bonus!).

It's unfortunate that in this world people are subjected to harassment and assault. But we can make a difference and help to make a change. To be an active bystander, the rule is if you see someone being harassed or assaulted, make your voice heard. You will be able to be an active bystander if you're aware of your surroundings. Always be alert and know what's going on. If you're in a situation and it feels "off," listen to your gut! Your instincts can help you understand whether something is wrong. Listen to your senses. Do you think you saw something or heard something? Then you probably did.

While witnessing assault and/or harassment can be scary, know that you *can* help! In fact, you're a critical part of helping to end assault and harassment. What you do *will* make a difference. But you also need to watch out for you, so it's important to be safe when you take action. When you intervene in a situation, make sure you're keeping yourself safe. It's better to deal with a dangerous or aggressive situation when you're with others. Get back-up, like from the police, by calling 911 if you see something. The police have training and know how to deal with aggressors, so it's okay to rely on them.

There are many people who are afraid to intervene in a sexual assault. Maybe they feel like it isn't any of their business. Maybe they are scared because they see something when they are doing something that they shouldn't be. Trust me, it's way more important to report a sexual assault than to worry about whether you're going to get busted for drinking underage or breaking curfew, or even for doing drugs.

Other things you can do, in addition to notifying the police or other authority, is to ask the victim if they are okay and let them know they have options (like going to a hospital if they are hurt or calling a hotline). You can also ask the person if they want to leave the situation. If it's a party, you can help them to secure a safe ride home. You don't have to be helpless when it comes to sexual assault. By being an active bystander, you *can* help.

Sadly, we live in a world where sexual harassment and sexual assault regularly occur and where sexually objectifying people is normal. But the more we talk about it and don't put up with assault and harassment, and the more we talk about gender norms and gender bias, the more we can change the world for the better. Get informed and get active. Changing the conversation is up to all of us.

19

WHERE CAN I GO TO GET MY OTHER QUESTIONS ANSWERED?

As we discussed at the beginning of this book, I don't have all the answers. And there is so much information out there to sift through and learn. What's real? What's fake? While this book is a general introduction to sex and sexuality and has a lot of information, at some point, you're going to want to know the answer to something that either I just introduced or I didn't talk about at all. Either way, you're going to need to look it up and the internet can be a great resource!

The challenge with online resources is that it's hard to know which sites are good and which sites are not so helpful. Also, a lot of times when you're trying to find answers and you enter something into your search browser, your search leads you to pornography, which isn't the best place to get answers about your sex questions. Why? Well, porn isn't really real. It's fantasy. Watching porn can set unrealistic expectations for yourself and/or your partner, or give you a false understanding of what sex and bodies are supposed to be like. It's much better to get your information from verified, factual sources. So, I've compiled some for you to go to, if and when you're ready. Sexuality is a lifelong journey. The types of things you like and don't like will probably change as you get older and yeah, old people have sex, but it's going to be different than 20-year-olds having sex. When you get to be a grandparent, you might need to look up some new things. I organized the sites by common questions to help start your further education. Again, these are sites that I know are medically accurate and designed for learning.

If you want more information on any of these:

- Is my body normal?

- Am I a virgin?

- Where can I find contraception near me?

- What contraception is best for me?

- Where can I get a STI test?

- Where can I get an abortion?

- Where can I get reproductive health care?

Check these out:

- Planned Parenthood is a great place to find lots of information! Start here: https://www.plannedparenthood.org/learn/teens and you can check out anything from questions about sex and your body to healthy relationships, what it's like to go to the doctor and how to keep yourself safe.

- Amaze is a great site that has a lot of animated videos that give real answers to all the questions you

have about sex, your body, and relationships. Go to
www.amaze.org to get started.

- Advocates for Youth is an organization that has lots
of information for teens, parents, and professionals with regard to topics of sex and sexuality. Go to
www.advocatesforyouth.org.

If you're curious about these types of questions:

- How do I know if I am gay?
- How do I "come out" to my family and friends?
- How can I stay safe if I am "out"?
- What do I do if I think I am transgender?

Then these are some great resources:

- GLSEN (Gay, Lesbian and Straight Education Network) is an organization that exists for students and
educators. This organization works to ensure schools
are safe for all youth.

- For general information and resources for youth,
check out www.sexetc.org. There is a lot of information there for teens ranging from challenging gender
norms, to information about sex, to how to get active in making positive change regarding issues like
school dress codes.

If you're in crisis, like you feel like you want to die, that things are hopeless or you want to kill yourself, these are great resources:

- The Trevor Project is crisis intervention and suicide prevention for LGBTQ youth. Go to www.thetrevorproject. org or call 1-866-488-7386 for help and resources.

- The National Suicide Prevention Lifeline is another great resource for youth (and anyone) in crisis. You can go to www.suicidepreventionlifeline.org or call 1-800-273-8255 for help.

- There's also the "It Gets Better Project" which is designed to help teens (especially LGBTQ youth) understand that while things are hard as a teenager, there is help available and that life *does* get better. You can go to www.itgetsbetter.org.

- Check out www.transyouthequality.org for more information and support if you are questioning your identity. This organization exists to support transgender and gender non-conforming youth, families and communities.

- Amaze has some great videos that address LGBTQ issues. Go to www.amaze.org to get started.

If you have relationship questions like:

- Is my relationship healthy?
- How do I know if I am in love with someone?
- What should I do if I am in an abusive relationship?
- How do I end an abusive relationship?

You should check out these resources:

- Love Is Respect is an organization with a 24/7/365 online chat program, a hotline and textline. You can learn all about different kinds of relationships and understand if your relationship is healthy and if it isn't, how to end it. Go to www.loveisrespect.org to chat or call 1-866-331-9474. TTY is 1-866-331-8453 and/or you can text "loveis" to 22522. The website is also available in Spanish.

- Planned Parenthood is a great place to find information on relationships. Check out this site: www.plannedparenthood.org/learn/teens/relationships for some basic information.

- Amaze has some cool videos about relationships. Go to www.amaze.org to get started.

If you have these types of questions:

- What do I do if I am sexually assaulted?
- Was it rape?
- How do I know if it's sexual harassment?

Check these resources out:
- RAINN is an organization that you can contact if you're in a crisis situation or for information and support. The website has tons of information about sexual assault, including rape, as well as sexual harassment. You can contact them 24/7 online through their online chatline at www.rainn.org or on their hotline which is 1-800-656-HOPE(4673). The website is also available in Spanish.

You might find you have the following questions:

- How do you engage in BDS&M?
- What is a fetish?
- Is what I like sexually a fetish?
- How do I act out fantasies?

Being curious about sexual behaviors and activities is totally normal. You might be curious about pleasure during sexual activity or interested in trying something a little different. Here are some great websites to look into less "mainstream" topics:

- www.bettersexed.org has a lot of information that you might be curious about but don't find on other sex education sites as it's focused on the pleasure aspect of sex.

Finally, if you're curious about statistics and laws, or have questions like:

- What are the laws of consent in my state?
- How many teens get pregnant in my state every year?
- How old do I have to be to have an abortion?
- How old do I have to be to get contraception in my state?

Check out these organizations:

- The Guttmacher Institute is an organization that does research in the field of sexual and reproductive health. Their website has information on laws as well as statistics that are really helpful. Go to www. guttmacher.org to find out about state-specific data and information.

- Power to Decide, formerly The National Campaign to Prevent Teen and Unplanned Pregnancy, is an organization that can help you understand how and where to access contraception, what laws are, and how to get active. They also have a lot of good statistics, infographics, and publications. To find this information go to: powertodecide.org/

The End?

And there you have it! You've been given the information and tools for "Making Sense of 'It.'" While the information in this book isn't everything out there regarding sexuality, I hope you've found it useful. Be safe and remember to communicate and advocate for yourself!

ACKNOWLEDGMENTS

Writing this book was a new endeavor for me and one of the scariest things I have ever done. All along the journey I had colleagues, friends, family and even strangers encouraging me. To the guy sitting next to me on the flight from Denver to Washington D.C.: Thank you for your awkward and gendered comments about pregnancy prevention for teens. Our conversation inspired me to rededicate myself to writing at a time when I was feeling pretty disillusioned with society after the 2016 election.

I'd also like to thank the awkward and inappropriate group of (what I assume were) coworkers at a wine painting party I happened to observe while I was in Albuquerque for work. The undertones of sexual harassment during those two hours of eavesdropping gave me the motivation I needed to finish the chapter on sexual harassment and solidify my instinct that ensuring young people understand consent and can define harassment absolutely belongs in this book. Sexual harassment and assault are not okay, and it's up to every single person to stop it.

I am so grateful for my Planned Parenthood training and education and the fact that I am able to help teens and parents have these important conversations! Before starting this book, the most I had written was curricula and presentations about sex and sexuality. There is no way I could have written this book without my formative experiences at Planned Parenthood. I also want to thank Planned Parenthood in their dedication to medically accurate and factual information. They were, obviously, a *huge* resource in making sure that all my deets were correct and up-to-date. I am forever grateful for *all* PP does for reproductive health—from education to medical services to advocacy. Planned Parenthood is a life-saving resource for so many millions of people across the country. Thank you for everything you do!

There are so many excellent leaders in the comprehensive sex education field that I am so grateful to. These organizations have helped develop me professionally, offered support to the content of this book, and helped inform the content. These amazing organizations are: Advocates for Youth, ANSWER, CARDEA, ETR, GLSEN, Healthy Teen Network, The National Campaign, Planned Parenthood, SIECUS, and the Trevor Project. Thank you, thank you for the work you do and the innovation and advocacy you lend the field. Additionally, I would like to thank the "Love is Respect" campaign and RAINN. All of these organizations work day in and day out to ensure that young people have the resources and information they need to make educated decisions about their lives. Thank *you*!

Specifically, I'd like to thank Leslie Kantor and Sonya Norsworthy at Planned Parenthood Federation of America as well as my colleagues from the different affiliates across the country—you know who you are! Your encouragement and mentorship over cocktails have meant the world to me.

I can't not give a shout out to my colleagues at Planned Parenthood of the Rocky Mountains, and especially those folks at the Responsible Sex Education Institute! These rockstar sexperts have been innovating and leading the field for years and I am so proud to be a part of this crew. There are so many people I have worked with and continue to work with who, without them, I would not be able to have written this book. So many people have cheered me on along the way: Marie, Adrienne, Julie, Persephone, Daniela, Elizabeth, Rosita, Brenda, Liza, Ryan, Becki, Brandi, Julissa, Dawn, Robert, Molly, Martin and so many more! Every day, these people change the lives of individuals in their communities. You are all truly inspiring and I am proud to work alongside you.

Finally, I want to thank all of my family and friends. Blake, Ben and Sam: you are my life, and I do what I do to try and make the world a better place for you. Thank you for encouraging me and believing in me. This book would not have been possible without your understanding and patience. Carissa, thank you for helping me to manage it all, even when I felt like I couldn't. Dad and Mom, thank you for instilling in me a passion for education and justice—it's the foundation for everything I do. Emgee, thank you for helping me shift negativity into positivity. Emily and Bert, thank you for being my biggest fans and helping me recognize that one person's voice can make a difference. Finally, thank you to my girlfriend crew and my mew crew. You ladies build me up and keep me going.